VETERINARY SCIENCES AND MEDICINE

REHABILITATING THE ATHLETIC HORSE

VETERINARY SCIENCES AND MEDICINE

Rehabilitating the Athletic Horse
Hank W. Jann and Bud Fackelman (Editors)
2010. ISBN: 978-1-60876-672-7

Veterinary Immunology and Immunopathology
Leon Neumann and Sophie Meier (Editors)
2010. ISBN: 978-1-60876-342-9

Veterinary Drugs and Growth-Promoting Agent Analyses
A. Garrido Frenich, P. Plaza-Bolaños, M.M. Aguilera-Luiz, and J.L. Martínez-Vidal
2010. ISBN: 978-1-60876-883-7

VETERINARY SCIENCES AND MEDICINE

REHABILITATING THE ATHLETIC HORSE

HANK W. JANN
AND
BUD FACKELMAN
EDITORS

Nova Science Publishers, Inc.
New York

For permission to use material from this book please contact us:
Telephone 631-231-7269; Fax 631-231-8175
Web Site: http://www.novapublishers.com

NOTICE TO THE READER

LIBRARY OF CONGRESS CATALOGING-IN-PUBLICATION DATA

Rehabilitating the athletic horse /Editors, Hank W. Jann and Bud Fackelman
ix, 222 p. : ill. ; 27 cm.
Includes bibliographical references and index.
ISBN: 978-1-60876-672-7 (hardcover)
1. Equine sports medicine. 2. Competition horses --Wounds and injuries --Treatment. I. Jann, Hank W. and Fackelman, Bud
SF956 .R44 2010
636.1 '08971027

2009044320

Published by Nova Science Publishers, Inc. ✢ New York

CONTENTS

PREFACE

This is a book about the restitution of soundness in horses which have been trained under seemingly ideal conditions, and nonetheless suffered injury. Most of the book's authors have had direct experience in performing medical and surgical interventions designed to correct athletic injuries. Most of the authors have also been directly involved in the conditioning techniques designed to not only render their own charges ready for competition, but also ready to win.

The book will suggest how things can "go wrong" even with man's best-laid plans. The text will then describe the path back from athletic injuries based upon that which is known about equine anatomy and physiology, and draw upon experience in human rehabilitation where applicable.

Some chapters will focus on how and when to apply therapeutic techniques, while others will describe in detail how, why and when those techniques are most beneficial. For instance, there are many measures which might be taken to treat a wound in such a way to enhance its healing, but have the psychological effects of relative isolation and inactivity shown to retard wound healing in laboratory animals, and almost assuredly operative in the healing of equine wounds, been considered?

It is anticipated this book will continuously evolve as even more is learned about the physiology of injury in horses and come to better understand how it might be prevented. For instance, what role does exhaustion play in the blunting of proprioceptive sense? The bones of a horse, when tested *in vitro*, can withstand any and all of the pressures theoretically placed upon them by running at speed. However, if no longer supported by a surrounding musculature, therefore loaded in unphysiologic ways, they fail. How can training for stamina at this basic levelbe better? There is hope to find out soon.

Chapter 1 - One of the driving principles of total rehabilitation is to maintain athletic conditioning while treating that which may be a serious, usually orthopedic, problem. While this ideal may not be reachable in some extreme cases, it *is* attainable in the majority of injuries the authors treat in the athletic horse. It usually means substituting another form of exertion for the one that caused the injury in the first place. In this way, the authors can avoid "de-training", from which it can be very time-consuming to recover. In arenas exemplified by, but certainly not limited to, our modern-day racing venues, three-day eventing, dressage and stadium jumping, such lost time can translate into considerable financial loss.

Alternative forms of exertion might include hand-walking, light riding, treadmills (dry or wet), or swimming. Any of these forms of exercise might be used to maintain cardiovascular fitness under strictly controlled circumstances. The selection will depend on the nature and degree of injury, its location, and economics. Local physical therapy (See Chapter 3) might include massage, range of motion (ROM) exercises, and alternating cold and warm compresses to reduce edema.

Chapter 2 - Physical activity places metabolic demands on horses above their basal metabolic rate, and successful adaptation to the desired physical activity is the result of both long-term and short-term changes in the horse's physiology that permit augmentation and reallocation of finite physiological resources. Acquired poor performance (distinct from failure to adapt to the desired exercise demands) results from an acquired defect in one or more organ systems that support exercise. This chapter will highlight the desirable adaptations that facilitate physical activity, the consequences of these adaptations on other physiological functions, and the approaches used to identify the defective organ systems that require rehabilitation.

Chapter 3 - This chapter deals with the special treatment of the injury for which the horse now finds itself in a rehabilitation program. As such, most of the methods described will be used in the early phases of the program, when healing of wounds, both surgical and otherwise inflicted will be of paramount importance. The authors will deal mainly with physical therapeutic measures and describe their practical applications. The subject of postoperative antibiosis has received ample coverage elsewhere [1], and will not be examined in any depth here. Regional physical therapy is directed at reduction of pain, avoidance of adhesions, and maintenance of a physiologic range of motion.

Chapter 4 - This chapter is an overview of two controversial therapies: stem cell and shockwave. The chapter begins by giving the reader a brief overview on the effects stem cells have on cells and the surrounding tissues. The author then explains the different types of stem cell therapies used in the horse and how they are collected and cultured. The stem cell section is concluded with case studies to describe how the author has used stem cells. The chapter flows into a brief description on how shockwaves are formed and transmitted. The chapter concludes with usage of the shockwave therapy for different conditions in the horse.

Chapter 5 - Five aspects of hyperbaric oxygen therapy are reviewed in this section; 1) the basic physical and physiologic principles that produce the desired increase in tissue oxygen concentrations, 2) the physiologic effects of hyperoxia, 3) indications for the use of hyperbaric oxygen as a primary or integrative therapy, 4) the potential application of hyperbaric oxygen in specific diseases including wounds, sepsis, bone healing and osteomyelitis, athletic injuries, reperfusion disease, blood loss, central nervous system diseases, carbon monoxide toxicity, 5) hyperbaric chambers and operation.

Chapter 6 - Within the last 25 years, the administration of medications directly into a joint has evolved into a skill and a mandatory procedure that nearly any equine veterinarian is expected to perform. The procedure has become an invaluable tool for the diagnosis, treatment and maintenance of joint health in horses used for any type of athletic use. The ever- increasing demands on such performance horses has produced a boon in our understanding of the pathophysiology of joint disorders in horses. As a result, the authors have seen an ever-increasing improvement in the specificity of therapy, and an increasing focus on joint health maintenance with Disease Modifiying Osteoarthritis Drugs (DMOAD), systemic medications and complementary therapies.

Chapter 7 - In addition to intra-articular therapies covered in a previous chapter, there are also a large number of other procedures that do not involve intra-articular injection. The goals of these therapies vary with the condition(s) being addressed, and as with intra-articular injection, the ability to meet these goals is heavily dependent on the completeness of the diagnostic approach and the accuracy of the diagnosis.

Chapter 8 - Although no conditioning strategy can be universally applied to all horses, there are some fundamental principles that should be followed when devising a conditioning strategy for a given individual. This chapter highlights the major concepts involved in conditioning a horse for competition and for reconditioning a horse during rehabilitation. The major focus is on developing a foundation and then adding to this with more intensified and specialized advanced forms of conditioning to develop strength, speed, stamina, and plyometrics. The concepts contained in this chapter can be applied to all equine disciplines.

Chapter 9 - The goal of this chapter is to increase awareness of the need for changes in how the authors view the success or failure of rehabilitation. By considering the psychological aspects of rehabilitation as well as surgery, wound treatment, and physical rehabilitation trainers begin treating each patient more thoroughly. Trainers will increase safety for horses and humans, reduce possible litigation for injuries occurring during rehabilitation, improve relations with clients and create confidence and assurance that trainers are treating someone's prized possession with the dignity, respect and care they deserve.

The mental and emotional aspects of rehabilitation are too often underemphasized or completely neglected. Horses in long term confinement situations often develop dysfunctional behavior patterns that can be difficult if not impossible to correct. This chapter is divided into four segments: 1) a typical case history 2) an explanation of why the mental and emotional aspects of equine veterinary care and rehabilitation can be problematic 3) specific mental and emotional aspects that must be considered during rehabilitation 4) and recommendations for improved care and increased success before, during and after the rehabilitation process occurs.

DEDICATIONS

To my father: A far better scholar than myself. He taught me how to hunt and how to work but never how to quit.

To Donna: Horsewoman, and healer of countless creatures both great and small. She personifies everything that is good about the veterinary profession.

The Village Blacksmith, Henry Wadsworth Longfellow:

Toiling, rejoicing, sorrowing,
Onward through life he goes;
Each morning sees some task begun,
Each evening sees it close;
Something attempted, something done,
Has earned a night's repose.
Thanks, thanks to thee, my worthy friend,
For the lesson thou has taught!
Thus at the flaming forge of life
Our fortunes must be wrought;
Thus on its sounding anvil shaped
Each burning deed and thought

Hank Jann

Special recognition to my daughter Paula F. Pierce and Dr Ann Kraus-Hansen for the efforts reviewing manuscripts and works in progress.

Bud Fackelman

ACKNOWLEDGMENT

Special thanks to John Bennett and Sarah Hill for technical and literary assistance with this work.

In: Rehabilitating the Athletic Horse
Editors: H. W. Jann et al., pp. 3-14

ISBN: 978-1-678-1-60876-672-7

Chapter 1

Overall Philosophy of Total Rehabilitation

G. E. "Bud" Fackelman
DVM, Dr med vet, DACVS, DECVS,
Oklahoma State University College of Veterinary Medicine,
Center for Veterinary Clinical Sciences, Stillwater, Oklahoma, USA

Abstract

One of the driving principles of total rehabilitation is to maintain athletic conditioning while treating that which may be a serious, usually orthopedic, problem. While this ideal may not be reachable in some extreme cases, it *is* attainable in the majority of injuries we treat in the athletic horse. It usually means substituting another form of exertion for the one that caused the injury in the first place. In this way, we can avoid "de-training", from which it can be very time-consuming to recover. In arenas exemplified by, but certainly not limited to, our modern-day racing venues, three-day eventing, dressage and stadium jumping, such lost time can translate into considerable financial loss.

Alternative forms of exertion might include hand-walking, light riding, treadmills (dry or wet), or swimming. Any of these forms of exercise might be used to maintain cardiovascular fitness under strictly controlled circumstances. The selection will depend on the nature and degree of injury, its location, and economics. Local physical therapy (See Chapter 3) might include massage, range of motion (ROM) exercises, and alternating cold and warm compresses to reduce edema.

Introduction

In any case involving a radical change in surroundings, the wise trainer will introduce the animal(s) to the exercise regime in a calm, carefully orchestrated, manner. Most horses will not have encountered some of the associated equipment, and may be intimidated by it. This must not be allowed to escalate to full-blown fear as this seriously prolongs the whole rehabilitation process. Slow, steady, quiet handling, possibly with the addition of mild tranquilization must be the rule. The presence of already acclimatized animals may also serve as a calming influence for "first-timers".

A program of gradually escalating levels of exercise should be conceived for each individual, and committed to paper. There should be goals set for each animal, and measurable outcomes predicted. Each animal must be evaluated as to the physiologic effects of the exercise program prescribed. This is most easily achieved by simply measuring pulse and respiratory levels before and after exercise. One rule of thumb is that 15 minutes of exercise (e.g. swimming) should elevate pulse and respiratory levels by 50%, and, that these levels should return to normal after 10 minutes of rest/ hand-walking. A lower value indicates that the exercise level is, *in this individual*, below his/ her current level of fitness, and its intensity and/ or duration may be increased at the next session. Higher values indicate the need to back-off and begin again more gradually.

Similarly, measurable goals should be set for the healing of any injury (ies). The measurements here might include surface area of a wound, degree of swelling, degree of pain on palpation, range of motion, degree of lameness, or radiographic or ultrasonic appearance [1]. Wherever possible, these values should be reduced to numerical terms (e. g., circumference, goniometric measurement, force plate analysis). In the absence of such numbers, regular photographic or cinematographic records can be used as alternative, minimal, measurements of progress. The use of either English or metric scales is a matter of personal preference, but whichever system is used should be consistent throughout any given facility. Deviating from such a plan only leads to confusion, and renders more difficult the comparison of responses between different individuals subjected to the same set of circumstances. When the treadmill is used as part of the rehabilitation program, it offers not only the ability to analyze gait, but also to evaluate upper respiratory function (via exercise endoscopy) and/ or vO_2 max [2].

The Administrator of a high-quality rehabilitation facility must assure that all records are filled-out clearly, at least on a daily basis, and that all diagnostic imaging (which chapters see) are of the highest quality. These records must not only be adequate for the ever-hopeful owner, but also be able to survive the scrutiny of any associated trainers and legal counsel.

IMPLEMENTATION

The first step in the rehabilitation of the equine athlete is to develop an exercise strategy that makes sense given the severity and character of its injury. It is better to err on the side of conservatism here, and to escalate the degree of exercise having observed the patient's individual response to your plan. Again, the protocol should be well thought-through, discussed with owners/ trainers, and committed to paper for all to consider. Then, the plan should be executed and carefully evaluated on a daily basis. Given that objective assessments (see above) remain positive, then the plan should continue to be pursued precisely as it was conceived. IF any changes are made, the reasons for those divergences from the original plan must be clearly articulated in the patient's record, along with a new set of measurements of progress.

For example, a given patient might have been scheduled for a daily regimen of underwater treadmill, dry treadmill, range of motion (ROM) exercises, and light exercise in hand or under saddle. IF during the ROM exercises, increasing pain were to be detected, then the second and fourth exercises mentioned might be curtailed or eliminated for several days, before being reinstituted at a lower level. At each stage in the progression of complete rehabilitation, the astute clinician must be prepared to retreat to a former level, and remain there until improvement appears before trying again. If that clinician is somewhat "removed" from the day-to-day operations, then (s)he must be especially careful in the selection of the individuals dealing directly with the animals, and have complete confidence in the validity of their observations.

STAFFING

This brings us to the most important consideration in the planning and realization of an effective Rehabilitation Center. Certain key individuals need to be on board during the planning and conceptualization of the Center, and ideally remain on-board to see their plans put into action. We have chosen to name these positions, ancillary to the actual clinical staff: the Medical Director, the Super Tech, and the Veterinary Technicians. Below, as examples, are the corresponding job descriptions prepared, based on previous experience, for a new facility in New York State (Courtesy of Juggernaut Farm):

Job Description Medical Director Nycart

The Medical Director (MD) is responsible for the overall management of performance, quality and service excellence at the New York Center for Animal Rehabilitation and Training (NYCART). These responsibilities include optimizing patient access and patient throughput, maintaining owner satisfaction, and operational effectiveness of the entire Equine and Canine Rehabilitation networks. Operations are managed through technicians and staff doctors assigned to each site.

Major responsibilities include, but are not necessarily limited to:

- Ensuring delivery of patient care in an environment that meets state-of-the-art standards, administrative best practices and service excellence.
- Establishing administrative protocols, workflow processes and procedures to optimize patient throughput.
- Ensuring that effective communication of the above protocols and adequate training is provided for all rehab personnel to ensure high levels of compliance.
- Regularly monitoring and taking corrective action, when required, through revisions and/or training activities.
- In collaboration with the NYCART Advisory Board and Owners, establishing annual performance indicators.
- Communicating annual goals and action plans down to front-line staff and monitoring those goals within all levels of personnel throughout the facility.

- Responsibility for measuring and reporting owner/ trainer satisfaction results and implementing corrective action plans based upon root cause analysis of key drivers of satisfaction indicators.
- Responsibility for the development of assumptions, communication and monitoring of the annual operating budget, ensuring labor and non-labor resources are appropriately allocated across disciplines in accordance with patient volume.
- Monitoring resource consumption trends and making adjustments throughout the fiscal year to ensure adequate labor coverage and supplies to meet key performance indicators.
- Ensuring adequate staff to provide impeccable maintenance of facilities and equipment, considering prevailing service levels.
- Tracking compliance with all local (Town of Stanfordville, Dutchess County, NY State), American Veterinary Medical Association, and Federal rules and regulations governing Animal Care Facilities.
- Collaborating with others as appropriate (e.g., referring practitioners, teaching institutions, breed associations, owners and trainers) to establish and monitor the delivery of high quality patient care through on-going assessment of clinical quality processes and improvement initiatives
- Providing first line response to physician and staff issues (behavioral and clinical).
- Responsibility for problem resolution, in collaboration with technical and professional staff as necessary.
- Fostering, developing and modeling professional excellence.

The successful candidate must be a seasoned leader with at least ten years' experience in direction and management of patient care. He/she must possess a veterinary degree, ideally be Board certified, and have demonstrated, through communication and publication, a keen interest in animal training and rehabilitation following injury. Experience should include exposure to optimization of patient throughput, owner satisfaction programs, and service excellence. Excellent communication, computer and financial skills are essential, along with an ability to translate goals into actions with measurable outcomes.

Job Description – Super Tech, Nycart

- Plans and administers medically prescribed physical therapy treatment for patients suffering from injuries, or muscle, nerve, joint and bone diseases, to restore function, relieve pain, and prevent disability:
- Reviews veterinarian's referral (prescription) and patient's condition and medical records to determine physical therapy treatment required. Tests and measures patient's strength, motor development, sensory perception, functional capacity, and respiratory and circulatory efficiency, and records findings to develop or revise treatment programs.
- Plans and prepares written treatment program based on evaluation of patient data.
- Administers manual exercises to improve and maintain function.

- Instructs, motivates, and assists patient to perform various physical activities, such as strength exercises, ambulatory functional activities, and use of assistant and supportive devices, such as casts, bandages and prostheses.
- Administers treatments involving application of physical agents, using equipment, such as hydrotherapy tanks and whirlpool baths, moist packs, ultraviolet and infrared lamps, cold laser, and ultrasound machines.
- Evaluates effects of treatment at various stages and adjusts treatments to achieve maximum benefit.
- Administers massage, applying knowledge of massage techniques and body physiology.
- Records treatment, response, and progress in-patient's chart and enters information into computerized record.
- Instructs owners and trainers in treatment procedures to be continued at home.
- Evaluates, fits, and adjusts prosthetic and orthotic devices and recommends modifications, if necessary.
- Confers with NYCART veterinarian(s) and other practitioners to obtain additional patient information, suggest revisions in treatment program, and integrate physical therapy treatment with other aspects of patient's health care.
- Orients, instructs, and directs work activities of veterinary technician(s), which job description see.
- May plan and conduct lectures and training programs on physical therapy and related topics for staff, students, and community groups.
- May plan and develop physical therapy research programs and participate in conducting research.
- May write technical articles and reports for publications or lectures at national level.
- May teach physical therapy techniques and procedures in educational institutions.
- May limit treatment to specific patient group or disability or specialize in conducting physical therapy research.
- Reports to Director of NYCART, and ultimately to the Senior Veterinary Consultant, the owners of NYCART, and its Board of Directors.

Individual positions will automatically have either a small or large animal focus, but successful candidates should be knowledgeable enough to be able to function temporarily in either discipline.

Job Description, Veterinary Technicians, Nycart

- Performs variety of animal health care duties to assist Veterinarian(s) or Physical Therapist(s) (Supertechs) in various NYCART rehabilitation areas (e. g., hydrotherapy pool(s), spa, treadmills, underwater treadmills, and hyperbaric oxygen chambers).
- Prepares treatment room for examination of animals, and holds or restrains animals during examination, treatment, or inoculation.

- Administers injections, performs venipunctures, applies wound dressings, cleans teeth, and takes vital signs of animals, under supervision of veterinarian or Supertech.
- Prepares patient, medications, and equipment for treatments, and hands instruments and materials to therapist(s) during various procedures.
- May perform routine laboratory tests, care for and feed animals, and assist professional personnel with clinical research projects.
- May assist veterinarian in the artificial insemination of animals.
- May bathe and groom small and large animals.

Routinely supervised by Supertechs (Physical Therapists), but may on occasion relate directly to NYCART veterinary staff or referring practitioners. Any direct communication with owners and/ or trainers should be OK'd by supervisor. Individual positions will automatically have either a small or large animal focus, but successful candidates should be knowledgeable enough to be able to function temporarily in either discipline.

Facilities

The Equine Rehabilitation Complex (ERC) planned for NYCART is a click or two beyond a state-of-the-art facility. The main building divides the stall section from the aquatics section. The twelve closest stalls are arranged in a half-moon design, which allows for easy observation from the centrally located office/lab area on the second floor. The aquatics section features two wash stalls with infrared warmers, the therapy pool, and underwater treadmill(s) (Figure 1). The HVAC in this area runs independently from that in the rest of the facility. This ensures appropriate temperature and humidity. Connected to the rehab barn by a covered breezeway and drive-through, is a 60ft x 130ft covered exercise arena, which also houses the hyperbaric chamber and treadmills (Figure 2).

Hyperbaric Oxygen Therapy has been shown to positively affect the healing of many tissues, including tendons, ligaments, bones, and vascular structures (see also Chapter 5). Above is an example of a unit designed to accommodate a horse (Figure 3). For our own facility, we have designed a special unit, that will not only accommodate several animals at once, but also lend itself to rehabilitate animals that are either paralyzed (e.g., botulism) or just in too much pain to bear weight on their limbs (e.g., laminitis or "founder"). For the latter cases we have designed a unique "Equine Gurney" that holds the animal suspended in a fitted girth and is propelled by a noiseless battery-powered motor. Below (Figure 4).

A covered breezeway, provides ramping to different floor levels between the structures, and can act as a loading/offloading area during darkness or inclement weather. Rehabilitating horses require that their physical activity be carefully controlled, but supervised relaxation ("down-time") is also important to the animal's psyche (see also Chapter 9). To this end, small turnout paddocks and "hot-walkers" are utilized.

The Canine Rehabilitation Unit is, in a way, a miniaturized ERC. It is housed at this particular facility in a 6700 ft^2, completely climate-controlled and soundproof underground bunker, originally designed as a bomb shelter (Figure 5). The inclusion of a canine unit on the same campus as its equine counterpart is a business decision based on sharing professional personnel, and better serving the clientele, most of whom own small animals as well as large, and are interested in optimal veterinary care of all of their charges. Thus, there is financial synergy between the two units producing a more viable enterprise overall.

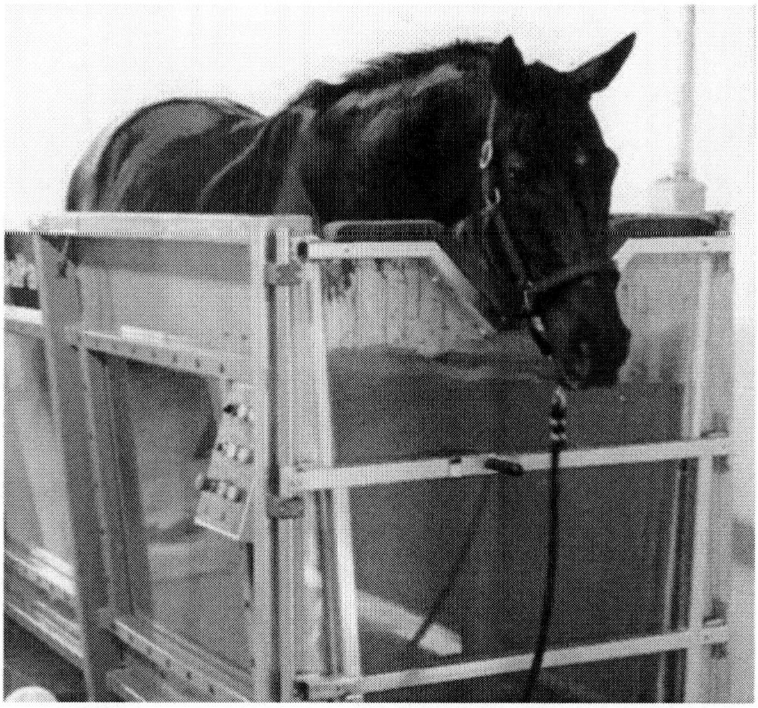

Figure 1. Equine Underwater Treadmill in action (Courtesy of Ferno, Inc.).

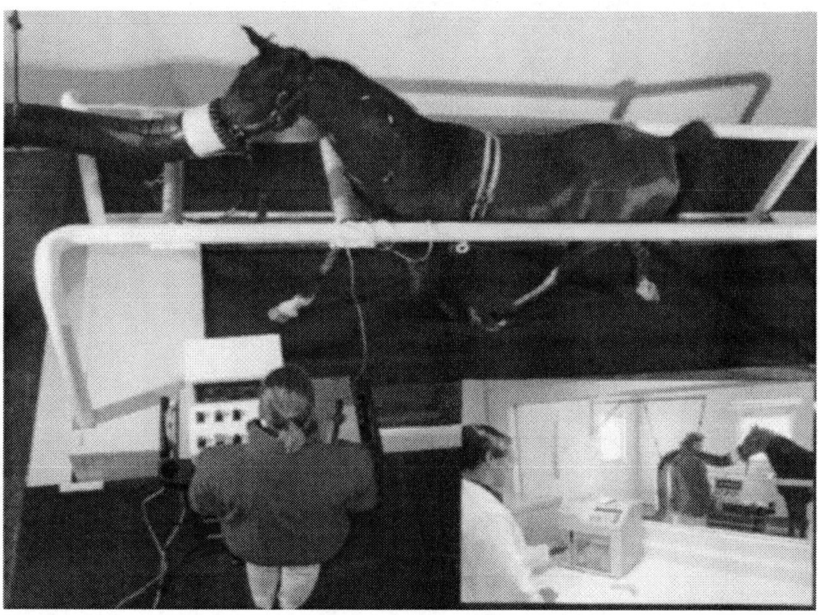

Figure 2. "Mustang" Dry Treadmill in use testing vO2 max as a measure of cardiovascular fitness. (Courtesy of Dr. Michael Weisshaupt, and Kagi Systems, Univ. Zurich).

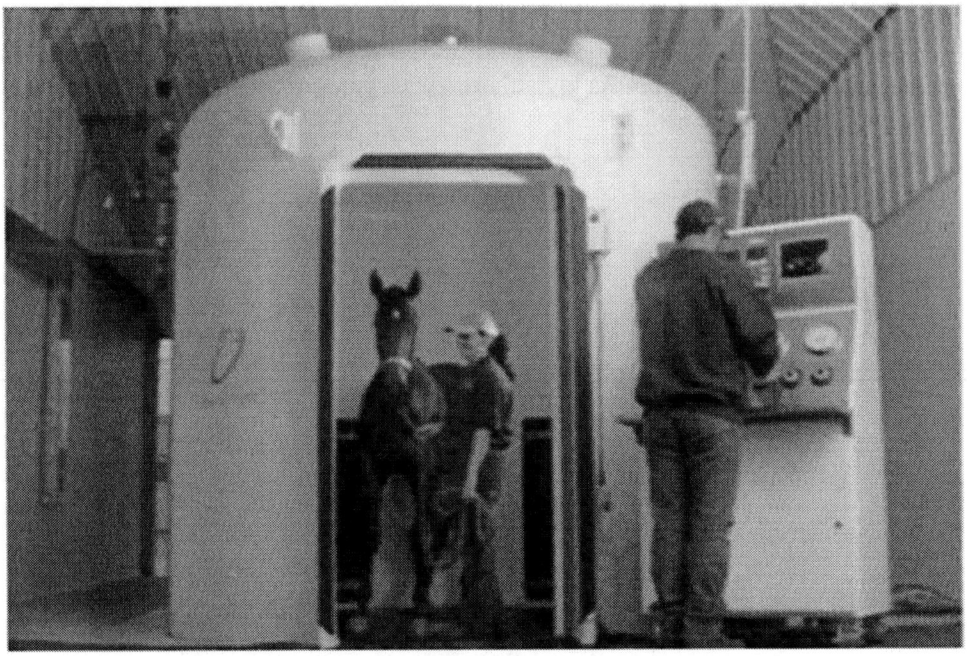

Figure 3. A Hyperbaric Chamber in use.

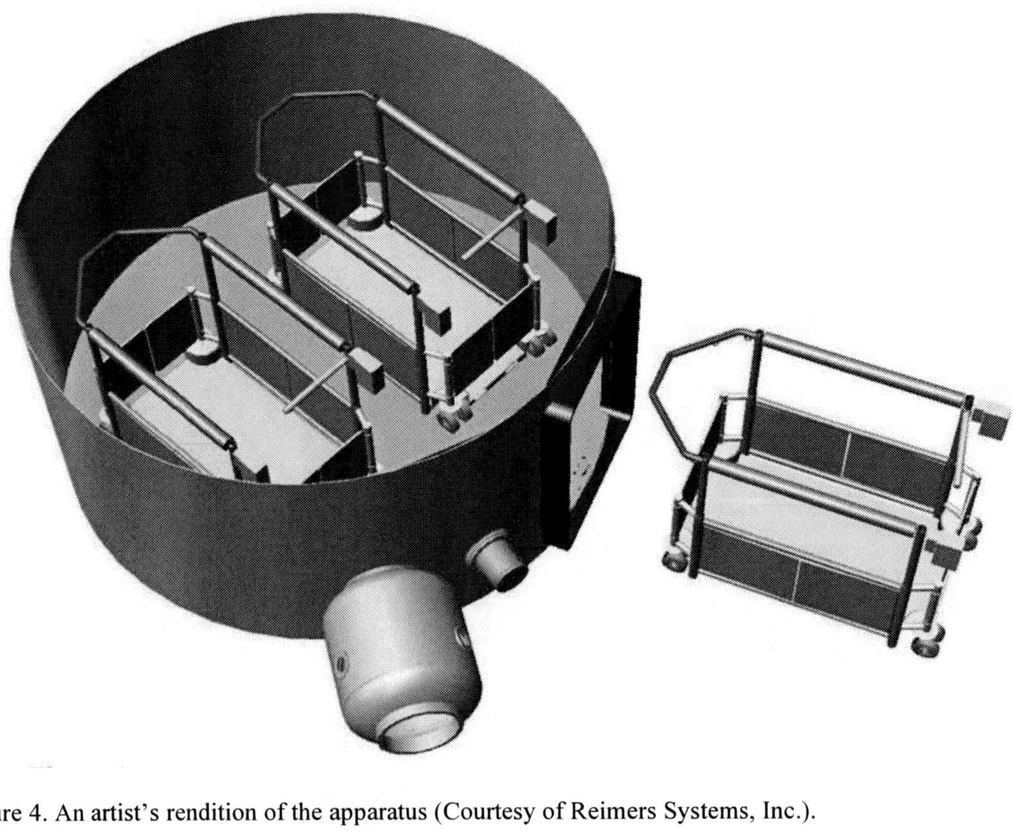

Figure 4. An artist's rendition of the apparatus (Courtesy of Reimers Systems, Inc.).

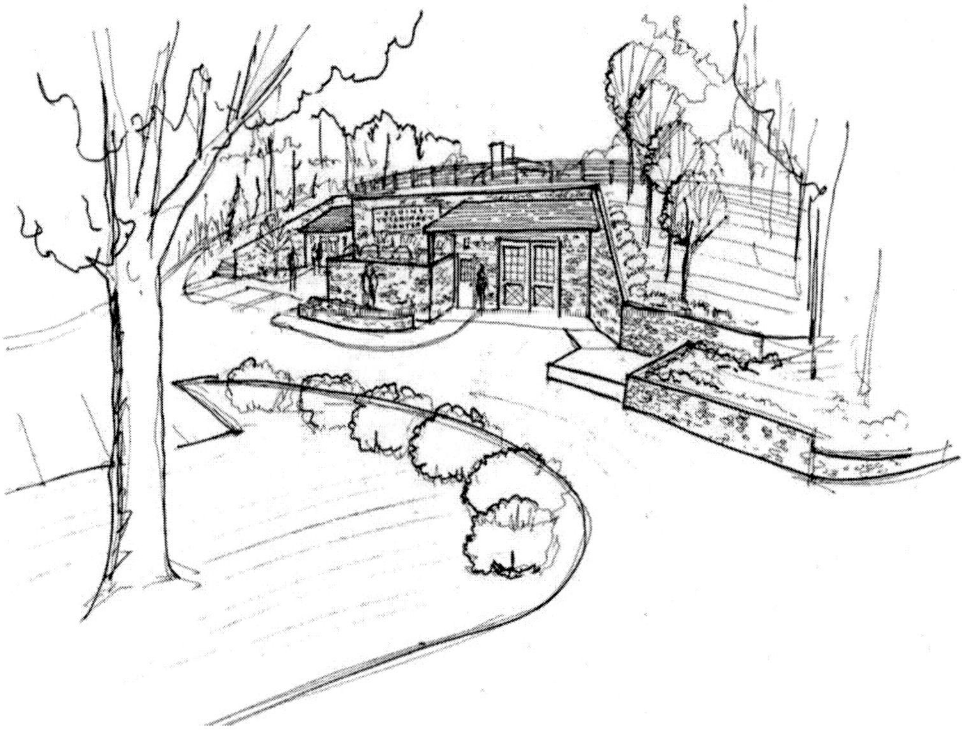

Figure 5. Entrance to the Canine Rehabilitation Unit.

Prior to treadmill exercise, many dogs receive analgesic cold laser or ultrasound (Figure 6).

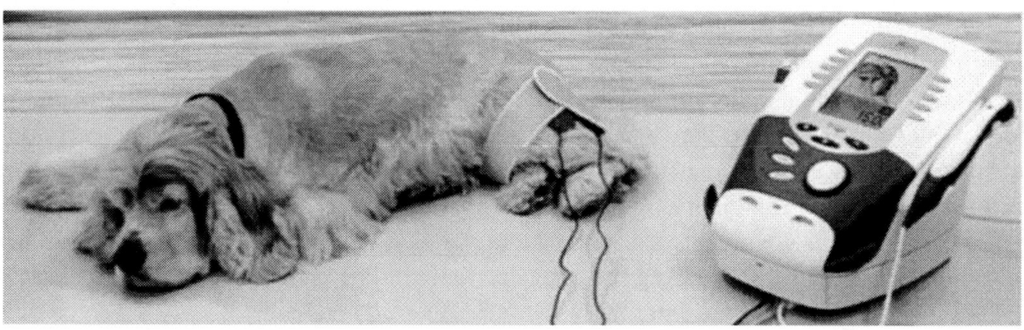

Figure 6. Dogs receive analgesic cold laser or ultrasound.

Some find the pain relief soporific. These patients may continue on to cardiovascular training in the swimming pool (Figure 7), joining those overcoming obesity, or others interested in additional conditioning for competition (agility, coursing, racing, etc.) There is space for housing convalescents over-night, or for longer periods.

Those readers interested in more information regarding Canine Rehabilitation should read, for starters, the book by Schulz et al [3].

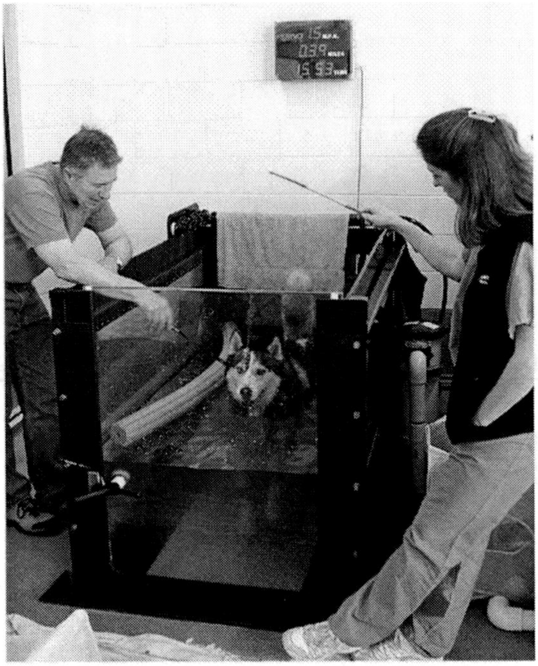

Figure 7. For postop small animal patients, the workhorse of the rehab unit is the underwater treadmill (Courtesy Alameda East Veterinary Hospital, Denver, CO.).

Discharge

Instructions given at the time of discharge from the rehabilitation facility are probably the most important factor effecting ultimate success in restitution of permanent soundness. Often they are glossed-over, or represent a "one-size-fits-all" reproduced set of orders that differ only slightly from one animal to the next. This is no longer acceptable.

We allot approximately an hour to the discharge interview with owner and trainer, and recommend that the entire conversation be recorded. A detailed Power Point presentation documents that which was performed on the animal in question, along with the dates and times of said treatments. The response of the animal to treatment is recorded, and any visual records produced to document that response are copied into the owners' set of documents. Before changing the subject during the conversation, all those present are asked for questions regarding material already presented.

We set up a schedule of reevaluations, and familiarize owners and trainers with e-report forms available on our web site, and how to complete and accurately transmit those forms. Any visits to the farm, ranch, or track are decided upon and committed to date books. Similarly, any anticipated needs for return visits to the Rehab Center are agreed upon and recorded.

We strive to objectivize the long-term evaluation of our treatment(s) via performance records available through, for example: the Jockey Club; trainers' notes; internet records of show results; or, club records of endurance/ competitive trail ride events. The owner is quizzed regarding appropriate channels for obtaining performance data, then *our staff* pursues those channels regularly. This responsibility cannot and should *not* be shifted entirely to the owner and/ or trainer. We consider it our job to verify that our ministrations were appropriate and effective – since, without that knowledge we are not really able to say we are "on the right track". Since this is a book about rehabilitating horses, the above objective performance parameters are limited to equine examples. Similar numbers are available online for the canine sector.

CONCLUSION

If all of the above seems to be a brave new look at managing injured animals, and trying to prevent re-injury, that's because it is. That a new look may be in order is certified by the fact that 700 – 800 racehorses are euthanized each year due to injuries sustained during competition [4]. In the face of a recent spate of breakdowns, a number of track sages have chosen to comment on the conformation of today's Thoroughbreds and especially on the "fineness" of their skeletal structure. They ignore the fact that numerous laboratories have shown that those bones are as strong as a similarly shaped structure made out of steel. However, even steel will fail if it is exposed to strain beyond that for which the part was designed.

An animal's (or a human's) skeleton develops according to the strain placed upon it. The strain increases or decreases dependent upon positioning. If a bone is repeatedly "bent" in one direction or another, internal remodeling takes place to reinforce the structure and make it strong enough to tolerate the new biomechanical situation. This takes place *gradually* during the training of any athlete, and is a matter of interplay between the skeleton and the musculotendinous structures that surround it. When this interplay becomes imbalanced, trouble ensues. As fatigue sets in, the muscle-tendon units are no longer capable of rapid or sustained contracture, and the bones' most important protective forces are stripped away. Added to that, the brain's perception of position in space (called proprioception) is also compromised. The human athlete gradually sinking into this state of affairs speaks of becoming "rubber-legged". The biggest differences between man and horse at this stage is that the former has no jockey urging him forward, and is not the herd animal driven desperately to stay with the pack.

We spoke earlier in this chapter of monitoring physiologic parameters (e. g., pulse, respiration) to determine degree of fitness, and, therefore, to increase or decrease levels of therapeutic exercise. Such monitoring plays a key role in conditioning endurance and competitive trail riding horses, whose running spans often 50-100 miles. Little or nothing of the kind is practiced during the typical training routine of the Thoroughbred racehorse. The speed with which a given horse can run 1/2 mile seems to be the only objective criterion regularly applied to measuring the degree of fitness [5]. Very few, if any racehorses ever experience running 1 1/2 miles (the Belmont distance, for instance) at flat-out speed prior to having to do it during the race. If the animal is "lucky" (s)he will be ridden by a jock that day that recognizes the problem, and will be "eased" as the saying goes. Disaster avoided, and, hopefully, training techniques might be altered to address the problem(s).

Another issue that can lead to negative consequences is the equivalent of the human quarterback's "playing hurt". There is an injury present (say, a knee problem) the pain of which the player can tolerate. He can pass, hand-off, avoid tackles, etc., but he is performing these maneuvers in an imperfect way (see John Madden's One Knee Equals Two Feet). Similarly, a large, heavy horse with a quarter-crack [6] might jog out "racing sound" on the morning of the competition, but be a "different animal" under the duress of a mile-plus competition. The natural rhythm of the gait becomes disturbed, cornering becomes more difficult, and all bets are off on which part of the musculoskeletal system will fail next.

Until we address Injury Profiling in racehorses more seriously, taking the entire animal and its training (or lack thereof) into consideration, we will not see any positive trends in the presently appalling euthanasia statistics. Fine boned? Ever seen the metacarpus of the world's second-fastest mammal: the Prong-Horned Antelope?

In summary, total rehabilitation of the equine athlete is complex, and many of the issues associated with it represent "moving targets" that demand close observations by experienced individuals if they are to be successfully resolved. The astute clinical staff- member and caregiver must observe the animals closely and become sensitive to their individual needs and responses. This is a very demanding endeavor requiring more than just "science", but it is an extremely fulfilling one when performed correctly. As more and more clinicians becoming interested in Total Rehabilitation, and, in the application of its evolving sports medicine, we can anticipate that more animals will be returning to their former levels of prowess, and fewer will be falling by the wayside – and that's a good thing!

REFERENCES

[1] Gillis CL. *Rehabilitation of tendon and ligament injuries*. Proc Amer Assoc Eq Pract, 1997:306-9.

[2] Gauvreau GM, Staempfli H, McCutcheon LJ, Young SS, McDonell WN. *Comparison of aerobic capacity between racing standardbred horses*. J Appl Physiol, 1995 Apr;78(4):1447-51.

[3] Schulz K. *The pet lover's guide to canine arthritis and joint problems*. St. Louis, Miss.: Saunders/Elsevier; 2006.

[4] Hodges CF. *Brief overview of trainer responsibility for racehorse breakdowns in New York*. Michigan State University College of Law The Animal Legal and Historical Center; 2008; Available from: http://www.animallaw.info/articles/qvusracehorsetrainer.htm

[5] Nafzger CA. *Traits of a winner: the formula for developing thoroughbred racehorses*. Neenah, Wis.: R. Meerdink Co.; 1994.

[6] Silberner J. *Bred for Edge, Greatest Racers May Have Handicaps*. All Things Considered, NPR; June 4, 2008; Available from: http:// www.npr.org/templates/story/story.php?storyId=91158342.

In: Rehabilitating the Athletic Horse
Editors: H. W. Jann et al., pp. 15-29

ISBN: 978-1-678-1-60876-672-7

Chapter 2

Exercise Physiology, Poor Performance, Overtraining

Michael S. Davis*

Department of Physiological Sciences, Oklahoma State University, Stillwater, Oklahoma, USA

Abstract

Physical activity places metabolic demands on horses above their basal metabolic rate, and successful adaptation to the desired physical activity is the result of both long-term and short-term changes in the horse's physiology that permit augmentation and reallocation of finite physiological resources. Acquired poor performance (distinct from failure to adapt to the desired exercise demands) results from an acquired defect in one or more organ systems that support exercise. This chapter will highlight the desirable adaptations that facilitate physical activity, the consequences of these adaptations on other physiological functions, and the approaches used to identify the defective organ systems that require rehabilitation.

Introduction

Exercise is, at a molecular level, nothing more than the conversion of chemical to mechanical energy at an accelerated rate. It is in this context that the optimal performance of exercise is best viewed, as it places nearly all the adaptations to exercise in their proper context. The adaptations of a horse to the performance of strenuous exercise can be divided temporally (i.e., short-term or long-term) or by the overall goal of the adaptation (increasing metabolic capacity vs. reduction of undesirable consequences). This chapter will outline the basic process by which physical exercise is achieved, identify the mechanisms by which the

* Contact Information: Michael S. Davis, DVM, PhD, Dipl ACVIM, Department of Physiological Sciences, Oklahoma State University, 264 McElroy Hall, Stillwater, Oklahoma 74078, Phone: 1-405-744-8172, Fax: 1-405-744-8263 Email: michael.davis@okstate.edu

capacity for physical exercise is increased, and characterize poor performance in the context of failure of adaptation to exercise.

SHORT-TERM ADAPTATIONS – THE TRANSITION FROM REST TO STRENUOUS EXERCISE DEMANDS OF MUSCULAR WORK

The process of extracting energy from complex macromolecules by biological tissues can be viewed as a whole as tissue metabolism, and skeletal muscle is the tissue with the greatest range of metabolism. Resting muscle consumes relatively little energy, whereas maximally exercising muscle can increase its metabolism 20 fold or higher. The processes collectively known as metabolism include substrate delivery, conversion of chemical energy to mechanical energy, and removal of waste products. Although these processes are highly coordinated and interrelated, it is useful to consider each individually before integrating them into the whole process of muscle metabolism.

Substrate Delivery

The basic substrates for the conversion of chemical energy to mechanical energy are oxygen and a carbon-carbon bond. Oxygen is not stored to a significant extent, and thus the muscle cell is completely dependent upon oxygen delivery through the blood stream. The source of oxygen is ambient air, and delivery accomplished through ventilation of the respiratory tract, diffusion into the blood stream, and transport through the cardiovascular system as oxyhemoglobin or, to a much lesser extent, dissolved oxygen. Although on a macroscopic scale this requires the expenditure of energy (in the form of cyclic contraction and relaxation of the diaphragm and heart), the movement of oxygen per se does not expend any energy. Rather, it flows down a concentration (partial pressure) gradient from the atmosphere to the mitochondia of the cell where it is ultimately burned. This point is critical, in that the flux of oxygen is entirely dependent upon the magnitude of the concentration gradient, and any stagnation of the transport system will result in rapid diminution of that concentration gradient, bringing the flow of oxygen (and therefore aerobic production of ATP) to a halt.

Supply of the carbon-carbon bond is dependent upon the identity of that carbon-carbon bond. Glucose can be supplied either from the bloodstream (arising from either dietary sources or hepatic gluconeogenesis) or through the breakdown of intracellular glycogen. Fatty acids are similarly supplied either from the blood stream (arising from dietary sources, adipose tissue) or from intramuscular lipid droplets. If the supply is delivered through the bloodstream, transport across the sarcolemmal is a necessary step that is a potential point of regulation for delivery of these compounds.

Conversion of Chemical to Mechanical Energy

Regardless of whether the glucose arises from the bloodstream or from glycogenolysis, complete metabolism begins with glycolysis, yielding a small amount of ATP and, more importantly, multiple 2 carbon acetyl groups that are completely oxidized through the Kreb's cycle and electron transport chain within the myocyte mitochondria. Fatty acids are broken down through beta-oxidation to 2 carbon acetyl groups that are similarly oxidized. Various points of these enzymatic cascades are regulated by substrate availability and energy needs of the cell.

A single muscle contains numerous individual cells, with potentially different metabolic capabilities. A basic criterion for classification is the type of myosin heavy chain within the cell, with the options of either Type I or Type II, with Type II further subdivided into Type IIA and Type IIX. Type I fibers are frequently designated "slow-twitch" fibers due to their slower cycling rate compared to Type II, or "fast-twitch" fibers. Combinations of these myosin heavy chain isoforms are also present within individual muscle cells, resulting in cells that can be characterized as Type I+IIA and Type IIAX. As a general pattern, Type I fibers also contain large numbers of mitochondria and thus relatively greater capacity for completely metabolizing macromolecular substrates into energy and terminal wastes. For this reason, Type I fibers are frequently termed oxidative (due to the large capacity to consume oxygen in the mitochondria) and fatigue resistant (due to the ability to produce large quantities of ATP). In contrast, Type IIX fibers contain relatively fewer mitochondria but large amounts of glycogen, permitting very rapid, but very short-lived production of energy even in the absence of oxygen. For this reason, Type II fibers are frequently referred to as "glycolytic" (due to the tendency to fuel contraction by the incomplete metabolism of glycogen) and "fatigable" (due to the limited amount of contraction that can be performed before fatigue). The "ideal" fiber (i.e., the fiber possessing the most robust capacities without shortcomings) is the Type IIA fiber. This fiber type possesses the capacity for rapid contraction along with high oxidative capacity.

Different muscles require different combinations of fibers, depending on the predominant activity of the muscle. In horses, the forelimbs are predominantly used for postural support, and therefore are comprised of Type I fibers that, although fatigue resistant, provide less power. Muscles of the hind limb provide the majority of the locomotor power, and thus are contain a higher proportion of Type II fibers. That is not to say that these muscles are exclusively Type II fibers. Rather, these muscle contain an oxidative core of fibers (Type I and Type IIA), with Type IIX fibers found in abundance in the more superficial areas of the muscle. This stratification is a critical consideration when performing muscle biopsies, as different regions of the muscle are activated at differing exercise intensities, and may have different responses to conditioning based on the pattern of activation as well as the original phenotype of the muscle fibers.

Removal of Wastes

The process of converting chemical energy to mechanical energy yields waste products that must be removed from the muscle, and ultimately from the body, in order for exercise to continue. The principle chemical wastes of complete substrate oxidation are carbon dioxide and water. Carbon dioxide is removed using the reverse process of oxygen delivery – that is, it is dissolved in blood, transported by the cardiovascular system to the lungs, and exhaled. The differences in physical chemical properties between oxygen and carbon dioxide are extremely relevant, though. As a molecule that can not only dissolve in water but also react with water, carbon dioxide is easily eliminated from the muscle. Excess carbon dioxide is also very easily cleared from the body through the lung, provided there is sufficient ventilation. This is not always the case in a maximally exercising horse, an idiosyncrasy that will be discussed later. Since carbon dioxide is a critical component of the body's systems for buffering pH, excessive elimination of carbon dioxide is undesirable and will cause dangerously high alkalinity in the body fluids. Elimination of water as a metabolic waste product is rarely a concern, since the body has an absolute requirement for water at rest, and this requirement increases during exercise due to the demands of heat dissipation.

The list of chemical waste products expands if exercise is supported energetically by anaerobic processes. Anaerobic metabolism to support exercise occurs when rate of initial breakdown of glucose exceeds the capacity of the mitochondria to fully oxidize the glucose to carbon dioxide. Although normal extracellular fluid contains approximately 85 mg of glucose per ml of fluid, uptake of this glucose into muscle is rarely rapid enough to exceed the oxygen delivery and utilization by mitochondria, and thus when extramuscular glucose is the sole source of glucose for energy metabolism, anaerobic metabolism rarely occurs. However, during periods of extreme demand, intramuscular glycogen can be broken down and produce glucose faster than can be fully utilized by the muscle. The initial breakdown of glucose can produce up to 6 mole of ATP/mole of glucose without the need for oxygen. The carbon-based end product of this reaction is pyruvate instead of carbon dioxide. If pyruvate is not further metabolized to carbon dioxide, as is the case with aerobic metabolism, then it is converted to lactic acid. Lactic acid is a potent organic acid that can lower pH and impair cellular function if allowed to accumulate. The body has numerous mechanisms by which lactic acid can be removed or converted back to pyruvate, but these processes have a low capacity and thus accumulation of lactic acid is a distinct possibility.

A final end-product of exercise metabolism, and one that is often overlooked, is heat. All reactions involved in the conversion of chemical energy to mechanical energy proceed down a thermodynamic gradient, and thus release energy in the form of heat. In fact, virtually all energy is eventually released as heat since only in rare circumstances is energy stored as potential energy (i.e., climbing and remaining elevated). If the exercise is relatively short, the generated heat is "stored" in the body through increasing body temperature, to be released into the environment after the exercise is complete. During maximal aerobic exercise, the metabolic heat production is sufficient to raise the body temperature of a horse by $1^{o}C$ for every minute of work unless heat is released into the environment. Although an equine athlete can tolerate a few degrees of hyperthermia for short periods of time, release of body heat is critical for horses exercising for more than a few minutes.

Metabolic heat is released through multiple physical processes, including conduction, convection, radiation, and evaporation. Conduction, or the physical transfer of heat from one substance to another by direct contact, is vitally important for moving heat generated in the muscle to the blood, and subsequently to the surfaces of the horse in direct contact with the environment. However, loss of heat from the horse through conduction is rarely a major contributor to overall heat loss due to the relatively low capacity of air for heat. (The exception to this statement is when the horse is bathed with cool water to accelerate cooling.)

Similarly, convection and radiation are not major mechanisms for heat loss. The major mechanism for heat loss is evaporation, either through the respiratory tract or through sweat. Respiratory heat loss is obligatory due to the absolute necessity of ventilation and the humidification of inspired air, and can account for up to 25% of heat loss. Sweating can account for up to 65% of heat loss in optimal conditions.

Regulation and Rapid Adaptation

In order to facilitate a 20-fold increase in metabolism, it is optimal to have the capacity to increase each of individual processes by 20 fold. On the other hand, maintaining that magnitude of delivery, conversion, and removal when it is not necessary (i.e., during periods of rest) would be extremely wasteful of the body's resources. The regulatory processes can be broadly divided into the processes that regulate the movements of oxygen and carbon dioxide, the processes that regulate the movement and storage of macromolecules used for energy, and thermoregulation.

Efficient movement of oxygen and carbon dioxide is achieved through control of the respiratory and cardiovascular systems. The amounts of oxygen and carbon dioxide in the blood stream are monitored individually by the brain, which increases the rate and depth of breathing based on decreasing amounts of oxygen or increasing amounts of carbon dioxide. A multitude of additional adaptations occur within the respiratory tract, including active dilation of the upper respiratory tract to reduce resistance to airflow and recruitment of secondary muscles of breathing to increase tidal volume and frequency. Typically, there is a slight lag in timing between the onset of exercise and changes in the blood concentrations of these gases due to exercise, so breathing is not immediately stimulated. However, the combination of high sensor sensitivity and a robust capacity for ventilation makes it possible for horses to closely control the blood concentrations of both oxygen and carbon dioxide during moderate exercise. However, during maximal exercise, fit horses routinely will demonstrate hypoxemia and, in extremely fit horses, hypercapnia. Exercise-induced hypoxemia in horses is the result of multiple physiological causes, including diffusion impairment, mismatch of ventilation to perfusion, and hypoventilation (when accompanied by hypercapnia). Hypercapnia is, by definition, caused by hypoventilation, which seems to be the result of expiratory flow limitation. That limitation does not appear to be due to the inability of the horse to generate more forceful expiratory efforts. Rather, the limitation appears to be somewhat voluntary – the horse elects not to direct the necessary resources (i.e., blood flow) to the respiratory muscles at the expense of locomotory muscles, and instead opts to accommodate the increase in carbon dioxide through buffering. Whether these deviations from normal blood gas values contribute to exercise limitation is not entirely clear, but recent data suggests that alleviation of exercise-induced hypercapnia will increase VO2, raising the potential for increased work prior to the development of fatigue.

Rapid adaptation of the cardiovascular system to changing exercise intensities (and by extension, energy demands of the muscle) is achieved on multiple levels. At the level of the working muscle, blood flow through the muscle is regulated by many individual valves within the capillaries. These valves open and close regularly, but the duration of their "open" conformation can be affected by the metabolic signals from the muscle. A decrease in the local oxygen concentration or pH, or an increase in local carbon dioxide or potassium (all consistent with contraction or increased metabolism) will result in greater percentage of the valve in the "open" position at any given time, thus increasing blood flow to the muscle cells. The increase in blood flow will increase delivery of oxygen, and increase removal of metabolic wastes (like carbon dioxide and organic acids).

The regulation of delivery of macromolecular fuel for muscle contraction is a much more complex process than the regulation of oxygen and carbon dioxide. The increased level of complexity arises from two properties of the macromolecules: The fact that they are not freely available, and the fact that they do not readily diffuse across cellular membranes. The former is addressed through storage and release of these molecules, both within the muscle and in other body tissues. The latter is addressed through specific transporters that facilitate the movement of these molecules across the muscle cell membrane. A limited amount of energy is stored in muscle, and thus very little exercise can be performed without movement of energy sources into the muscle. Stored ATP can fuel just a few contractions of muscle, and intermediate energy storage molecules, including intracellular glucose, fatty acids, and their intermediate breakdown products can provide 15-30 seconds of maximal contraction. Any further work must be supported either by breakdown of intramuscular macromolecular stores or transport of glucose and/or fatty acids from the bloodstream into the muscle, and the processes that permit increased availability of macromolecular energy to the muscle cell are critical adaptations that permit exercise. Moderate levels of exercise are supported through the use of relatively abundant extramuscular substrates (in preference to the more finite stores of intramuscular substrates). Muscle contraction stimulates the movement of substrate transporters onto the sarcolemma to facilitate transport of glucose and long-chain fatty acids into the sarcoplasm. In the absence of these transporters on the cell surface, very little glucose and fatty acids can be transported into the cell, making movement of these transporters a critical feature of sustained exercise. Breakdown of intramuscular stored macromolecules (fat and glycogen) occurs when the energy state of the muscle cell begins to drop despite the recruitment of glucose and fatty acid transporters. When the amounts of ADP and AMP increase within the cell, selected enzymes are activated that breakdown intramuscular glycogen, releasing glucose within the cell to be used as energy. A similar process occurs with respect to intramuscular fat, producing fatty acids. Just as important, decreases in the energy state of the muscle activates genes to stimulate the production of more energy-harvesting enzymes and transporters. This sequence of priorities is important in two ways: First, by placing a priority on use of whole body stores (as opposed to internal stores), the horse maximizes its overall exercise capacity; and second, in order to increase the exercise capacity of the muscle, it is necessary to work it hard enough to create an energy deficit, thus stimulating the cell to produce greater capacity.

The concentrations of glucose and fatty acids circulating in the bloodstream must be maintained as the exercise-stimulated transport into the muscle increases. Maintenance of blood glucose and fatty acid concentrations is achieved by hormonally-mediated release of these compounds from storage sites within the body. Glycogen and fat are the primary storage forms of glucose and fatty acids, respectively. When these nutrients become available in excess of demand, such as immediately following ingestion of a meal, the body releases insulin to facilitate storage of the excess energy nutrients. During exercise, most horses will experience a decrease in circulating insulin concentration and an increase in circulating glucagon concentration. The combination of these hormonal changes will permit the release of fatty acids from fat stores (insulin drop) and stimulate the release of glucose from the liver, either due to breakdown hepatic glycogen or conversion of certain amino acids to glucose (glucagon rise). Under resting conditions, insulin is needed to activate macromolecular substrate transport into muscle cells. However, during exercise the lack of insulin is compensated by the previously-described effect of contraction on substrate transport. Glucocorticoids may also play a role in maintenance of energy supply to the muscle by stimulating protein breakdown and liberation of amino acids for gluconeogenesis.

LONG-TERM ADAPTATIONS – THE EFFECTS OF CONDITIONING

Conditioning for exercise performance follows the general principles of stress, strain, and remodeling. (Throughout this chapter and most texts on exercise physiology, conditioning is defined as the physiological adaptation to increase exercise capacity, or the activity that produces those physiological adaptations. Training is the mental process of learning a particular activity, behavior, or response.) Stress is the application of force to a system, strain is the resulting deformation, and remodeling is the change in the system that is stimulated in response to the stress-strain episode. In an ideal system, the remodeling results in reduced strain for a given stress. Conditioning is thus the catch-all term for the entire panoply of systems remodeling in response to repeated exercise, and is distinct from the short-term adaptations previously described in that conditioning is the result of quasi-stable changes in the systems.

A critical principle of athletic conditioning, regardless of the species or discipline, is that conditioning is activity specific. The body seeks efficiency in the use of energy and nutrients, and since the physiological changes that comprise effective conditioning require both energy and nutrients, the body will not increase the capacity for exercise unless such increase is clearly needed. In other words, some degree of physical or metabolic stress is required in order to stimulate conditioning. The stress need not be enormous, and in fact too much stress can result in damage to the stressed tissue, resulting in injury and impeding conditioning. It is also important to recognize that a tissue that is not stressed will not adapt. Thus, if conditioning does not closely mimic the desired activity, some or all of the tissues needed to perform the desired activity will not be conditioned to a higher level of performance and will thus be the limiting factor(s) in exercise performance.

Skeletal

The clearest example of the role of stress and strain in the process of exercise conditioning can be seen in the adaptation of the skeleton to exercise. Even during sedentary existence, all portions of the skeleton are subject to a modest range either compressive or distractive stresses (depending on the specific location), but undergo minimal strain due to the construction of the bone in those areas. During locomotion, the range of stresses increases and with those increases comes greater strain, resulting in modeling (reshaping due to the addition of new bone) and remodeling (reshaping due to bone turnover) in a process known as Wolff's Law. The intended and logical goal of the modeling process is to decrease the strain associated with the new stresses, thus preserving the structural integrity of the bone.

It is intuitively obvious that the magnitude of stress increases with increasing speed, and this belief is supported by objective research. Pure vertical stress nearly double in transition from walk to canter, and forward stresses can more than double. The resulting strain on the dorsal metacarpus increases 6 fold from a walk to run in mature horses. What is less intuitive is that the direction and distribution of the stresses changes with changing gaits, resulting in distinct patterns of strain. These observations highlight the importance of specificity of adaptation – trotting will produce a characteristic pattern of strain, and the resulting adaptation will be optimized for resisting the stresses of trotting, but not necessarily another pattern of loading (i.e., another gait).

The precise manner in which strain is detected and transduced into signals for osteoid deposition or resorption is currently unknown, but the most popular hypothesis has identified the osteocyte as the cell that is responsible for this transduction. Rather than being a discrete cell isolated within osteoid as was once thought, osteocytes possess long dendritic processes that permit direct contact with both the surface of the bone as well as the marrow, thus permitting the osteocyte to communicate directly with osteoblasts and osteoclasts in the active regions of the bone. Loading of the osteocyte (or of the osteoid surrounding the osteocyte) is likely detected by deformation (strain) of the dendritic processes of the osteocyte, and results in secretion of DMP1, which stimulates mineralization of osteoid. In contrast, unloading of the osteoid results in secretion of sclerostin, which inhibits osteoblasts. Thus, the net change in mineralized osteoid is the result of the balance between these chemical signals. With exercise, increased strain results in increased osteoid, providing structural resistance to strain and eventually returning to a balanced signal. The major practical point of this process is that load is an absolute requirement for modeling, and modeling is an extremely local phenomenon, controlled by individual cells. It is also important to note that only a few characteristic loading cycles are required to stimulate the modeling process, and the application of additional cycles after the modeling process has been activated do not further the process.

Cyclic application of stress produces cyclic strains, and the degree to which the material recovers from those strains is a critical feature of whether failure is likely to occur. If the material returns to its previous state, elastic deformation is said to have occurred. If, however, the material does not return to its previous state, then plastic deformation is said to have occurred. The application of these terms to a biological system is treacherous due to the nature of the system and the problem of defining a complete return to the previous state, but it is sufficient to suggest that a certain degree of plastic deformation is both permissible and desirable, insofar that the plastic deformation is defined by a change in osteocyte activity that leads to the production of stress-resistant bone. The development of microcracks is another, more severe form of plastic deformation. Initially, microcracks will change the structural properties of the bone, increasing the strain (deformation) produced by a given stress. Although these structures may have a initial beneficial role by absorbing energy without catastrophic failure, they are also likely to accumulate and permit progressively greater degrees of deformation, ultimately leading to fatigue and failure. The possible fates of the microcracks are two-fold. The majority of microcracks probably heal by remineralization, evidenced by the abundance of these structures in post-mortem bone samples collected from sound horses. However, resorption and remodeling is another possibility. Initial resorption removes matrix and further weakens the bone. Although, this process appears to be inhibited by the sustained loading seen in routine training, such inhibition can be removed by a break in routine loading such as temporarily being removed from training. This process is hypothesized to be the underlying cause of catastrophic failures that occur when a horse is returned to racing after a short lay-off.

Tendon

The perception of tendon as a dynamic, adaptable tissue is a relatively new concept, but one that is borne out by recent research. In longitudinal studies of Warmblood foals, subjects that were permitted unrestricted exercise in pasture had larger, stronger, and better quality tendons at 5 months of age than subjects that were either confined to box stalls for the duration of the study, or confined to box stalls but treadmill exercised during the study. More importantly after all foals were turned out, there was limited (incomplete) recovery of tendon metabolism in the boxed foals relative to the pasture foals at 11 months of age. Similar findings were reported in a study of Thoroughbred foals, with the additional observation that treadmill exercise in addition to pasture exercise did not substantially improve tendon properties over pasture exercise alone.

The findings of tendon conditioning in foals are in stark contrast to studies of the effects of conditioning in older horses (> 2 yrs old). Aging is associated with changes in morphology, composition, and metabolism that reduce tendon strength, and these changes are accelerated with the superimposition of exercise. Collectively, these studies lead to the conclusion that there is a narrow window of adaptability of tendons, beginning and birth and ending at approximately 2 years old, possibly sooner. These findings underscore the importance of very early exercise in the production of tendon that best suited for a lifetime of exercise.

Cartilage

Evidence for long-term cartilaginous adaptation to exercise is sparse, but it is safe to conclude that appropriate conditioning (i.e., conditioning that does not injure the cartilage) will improve its ability to function under the higher loads of exercise, provided this conditioning is applied while the cartilage is metabolically malleable. Similar to tendons, equine cartilage appears to be most adaptable during immaturity, and there is little evidence that changes that occur in response to training of mature horses are beneficial. In foals, exercise readily produces an increase in cartilage content of glycosaminoglycans, presumably increasing the capacity for impact absorption and joint lubrication. In 2 year old horses, one study of high intensity training can result in increased cartilage thickness, but may also result in increased degenerative changes. In contrast, another study of trained 2 year old horses found increased thickness of hyaline cartilage with no pathological changes. A major difference in study methodology (treadmill vs. track training, respectively) may help explain these differences, but the overall paucity and conflicting information regarding cartilage adaptation in older horses warrants caution in concluding that cartilage can be favorably adapted in horses undergoing formal athletic training.

Muscle

Muscle is the tissue that is probably the most readily adapted to exercise, and the obvious increase and toning of muscle mass in response to conditioning is the easiest adaptation to detect. However, the visible muscle changes are not the only adaptation that occurs in response to conditioning. Changes in fiber contraction speed, metabolic capacity, metabolic strategy, and capillary density all can occur in response to conditioning, with the overall goal of improved muscle performance. Changes to the muscle are specific to the type of activity that stimulates the change – activities that emphasize explosive power, such as sprinting and jumping, tend to produce muscle with increased power, whereas activities that emphasize fatigue-resistance, such as endurance racing, tend to produce muscle with greater capacity for sustained contraction. It is important to note that as a general statement, these types of muscle are mutually exclusive. That is, muscle with high endurance capacity does not generate as much explosive power as muscle designed for that purpose, and vice versa. This phenomenon underscores the importance of specificity of training in building the appropriate muscle for the intended activity.

The increase in muscle mass resulting from conditioning is produced through either hypertrophy of individual muscle cells, hyperplasia of the muscle cells, or a combination of the two. Muscle hypertrophy, or increased size of individual muscle fibers, has been reported in response to power training, such as jumping or sprinting. The primary disadvantage of fiber hypertrophy is the obligatory increase in diffusion distance between the muscle fibers and the capillaries, making these fibers more prone to fatigue during prolonged work at peak capacity. This disadvantage is of minimal concern if the anticipated activity is very short and can be supported through glycogen breakdown and/or anaerobic metabolism, but is undesirable for longer activities. In contrast, increased muscle mass due to fiber hyperplasia may not have as many power-generating units (actin/myosin crossbridges) per cross-sectional area, but the "missing" power-generating units are replaced by a denser network of capillaries that more efficiently supply exogenous substrates and remove wastes generated during exercise, thus making the muscle more fatigue resistant. Muscle fiber hyperplasia is the predominant mechanism of increased muscle mass in not only endurance horses, but also most racing Thoroughbred and Standardbred horses.

Conditioning causes changes in overall fiber types, with a progressive shift from fast-twitch, low oxidative fibers (Type IIX) to fast-twitch, high oxidative fibers (Type IIA) and further to slow-twitch Type I fibers. The shift from Type IIX to Type IIA appears to be readily accomplished with virtually any type of conditioning program, with the possible exception being very intense, short-interval regimens that may permit a decrease in Type I fibers. Shifts towards Type I fibers are generally accomplished with prolonged training regimens. Concurrent with the shifts in fiber types comes an increase in oxidative machinery and the capacity for transport of substrates across the sarcolemma. Finally, aerobic conditioning is associated with increased capillary density, a feature that permits more rapid diffusion of substrates and wastes into and out of the muscle during exercise.

Cardiovascular

Cardiovascular adaptations are the most prominent adaptations resulting from effective conditioning, and generally contribute the greatest to increased exercise capacity. Cardiovascular adaptations fall into 3 general categories: Heart, capillaries, and blood volume. The primary direct effect of conditioning on the heart is cardiac hypertrophy, or enlargement of the heart. Not only is there more heart muscle, but the chambers of the heart are also larger. The combination of these two changes results in much more effective pumping of blood, a greater capacity for cardiac output during exercise, and a much slower heart rate at rest. The normal resting heart rate of a horse is 40-44 beats per minute, but it is not unusual to find conditioned horses with hcart ratcs below 40 beats per minute. Very well conditioned horses may even present with intermittent dropped heartbeats, as the heart rate slows so much that the ventricles do not contract with every electrical impulse. In fact, decreasing heart rate in response to conditioning is a predictable enough response that many trainers will use the resting heart rate of their horses to gauge the effectiveness of their conditioning regimen.

Increased blood volume is a second, very common change associated with exercise conditioning. The mechanisms of blood volume expansion are not entirely known, but overall, blood volume expansion is the result of fluid retention by the kidneys through conservation of sodium. To the extent this action is driven by release of aldosterone, sodium retention may come at the expense of potassium conservation, potentially leading to a whole-body deficiency of potassium. Potassium deficiency is a potential contributing cause to some exercise-related disease syndromes, to be discussed later in this chapter. Although there is greater blood volume, blood pressure does not necessarily increase since veins will expand to accommodate the additional fluid. When needed, the veins can constrict, increasing the pressure in that segment of the circulation and facilitating faster filling of the heart.

Increased density of capillaries in the muscle is a third area of cardiovascular adaptation to exercise, but one that is the least studied. Most scientists assume, based on mathematical models, that the muscle develops more capillaries in order to more effectively transport gases, substrates, and heat during exercise, and there are some studies that support these beliefs. However, due to the technical difficulties inherent in these studies, they are limited. From a practical standpoint, the importance of increased capillary density in the muscle of exercising subjects is best illustrated by the artificial effects of some drugs on muscle. If muscle mass is increased through drug use, but is not accompanied by increased capillary density, the muscle effectively becomes excess weight and overall athletic performance decreases (despite the subject being “muscled up”).

Respiratory

The respiratory system displays minimal adaption in response to conditioning, in stark contrast to most other systems involved in exercise. Multiple longitudinal studies have failed to detect increases in tidal volume or ventilatory flow rates independent of the effects of growth. Rather, conditioning is associated with greater severity of hypoxemia and hypercapnia at maximal exercise (albeit at greater absolute levels of exercise compared to pre-conditioning) as the rest of the horse develops a greater capacity for exercise. These findings underscore the fact that as the likely organ system ultimately responsible for the greatest limitation to exercise, any abnormality of the respiratory tract is almost certain to contribute to impaired performance.

Deconditioning

The maintenance of conditioning adaptations generally requires the activities that initially stimulated the adaptation. As a general rule, the various tissues and systems that adapted to exercise will return to their pre-conditioning state with rest of sufficient duration in a process known as deconditioning. Deconditioning is an important physiological phenomenon because athletes invariably have their activities interrupted for various reasons ranging from illness and injury to management issues, and the horseman must be aware of the extent to which critical systems may no longer be adapted to the desired level of exercise.

The knowledge base of equine exercise physiology is incomplete with respect to patterns of deconditioning and methods for minimizing the loss of conditioning during periods of rest, but there is enough information available to draw some conclusions. The more readily adapted tissues appear to also be the tissues most susceptible to deconditioning. Bone mineral content is largely preserved up to 3 weeks of deconditioning, but then begins to decrease rapidly. This effect can vary with different areas of the skeleton, with some areas preserving bone mineral content up to 9 weeks. However, in the same way that a chain is only as strong as its weakest link, the portion of the skeleton that loses its strength the fastest must be considered the most relevant for the effects of deconditioning and preservation of exercise capacity. Deconditioning of cardiac performance appears to be similar to that of bone, with cardiac mass and performance maintained for up to 4 weeks of inactivity before decreasing precipitously. Conditioned muscle can be expected to retain its adaptation to exercise for up to six weeks of inactivity, but will almost completely detrain after 12 weeks. Changes in muscle fibers during detraining are simply the reversal of the training pattern – the muscle gradually replaces Type I fibers with Type IIA fibers, and then Type IIB fibers. Parallel changes in oxidative capacity and fiber size also occur.

Despite these changes, aerobic capacity is well preserved during the initial phases of deconditioning. Studies have found minor decreases that did not achieve statistical significant after 12 weeks of rest, although the general trend for decreases maximal oxygen uptake is clearly visible on the plotted data. The lack of statistical significance may reflect the higher technical variability in these measurements compared to other indices of conditioning.

Physiological Basis of Poor Performance – Failure of Adaptation

Poor performance is a common complaint in equine athletics, and often it is up to a veterinarian to determine the cause and possible remedy that will restore performance. The physiological basis for poor performance can be reduced to three broad categories: Failure to condition, acquired defects, and overtraining.

Failure to condition is probably the most common cause of poor performance, and also one of the most frustrating for a diagnostician. Included in this category are horses without the genetic capacity to reach the desired level of performance, as well as horses with training regimens that are inappropriate or insufficient for the desired performance. Merely the fact that a horse has been exercised does not constitute proof that a horse has been conditioned, or that the conditioning that has occurred (if it indeed occurred) was appropriate to improve performance. Perhaps the best single clue for determining whether poor performance is related to failure to condition is the answer to one simple question: Has the horse EVER performed at the desired level? If not, then a close examination of the conditioning program and evidence for an expected physiological effect of that program is in order. If so, then it is rational to consider other physiological causes of poor performance.

Acquired defects that cause poor performance can affect nearly every system in the body, but not every abnormality found in an equine athlete can be credibly blamed for poor performance. Rather, the diagnostician must consider the demands and necessary adaptations of each body system that facilitate the desired performance, and how a particular abnormality might interfere with those adaptations. For example, sprinting performances (activities lasting less than 20 seconds) are not highly dependent upon the ability to remove wastes from the body due to the capacity to temporarily store these wastes without affecting performance. Thus, it is unlikely that impaired sweating would lead to poor sprinting capacity. Conversely, performance in a race lasting 2-5 minutes is highly dependent upon the ability to transport oxygen to the working muscle, and any abnormality that decreases oxygen uptake and delivery can be expected to impair performance. In most cases, the relationship between the acquired abnormality and the physiology of poor performance is less obvious than the examples provided, but these examples serve to illustrate the general requirement for considering the physiology of the desired performance when evaluating an athlete for poor performance.

Overtraining is a third potential cause of poor performance, and one that has only recently been characterized in an objective manner. The term "overtraining" originated in human exercise physiology, and has been loosely defined as a long-term (> 2 weeks) decrement in performance without relevant physiological symptoms. Such a definition is obviously subject to abuse, since the conclusion that there are no relevant physiological symptoms often depends on the rigor with which one looks for those symptoms. Indeed, the recent advances in research into overtraining in both humans and horses serve to make the very concept of overtraining obsolete, since these advances have defined a specific physiological phenomenon characteristic of "overtraining" that can rightfully be considered as no more than an acquired condition that results in poor performance.

Overtraining must be distinguished from excessive training intensity (overreaching) or inadequate metabolic recovery. In the case of the former, exercise intensity that overwhelms the musculoskeletal systems may present as an unexplained loss of performance, when in fact the loss of performance is due to musculoskeletal damage that is not permitted sufficient time to heal between exercise sessions. Overreaching may not lead to overt clinical signs of lameness or muscle soreness, but closer examination of the horse will disclose occult muscle, tendon, joint, or bone damage. Inadequate metabolic recovery is similarly an imbalance between exercise and recovery, but on a milder scale. Like most athletes, horses rely on intramuscular macromolecules to fuel strenuous exercise, and these reserves are prone to depletion. Horses are relatively slow to replenish these reserves compared to other athletic species, and without repletion, the horse will have less capacity for endurance at the levels of exercise that require intramuscular oxidative substrates.

A neuroendocrine basis for overtraining is likely. Strenuous exercise generates physiological stress, and a transient increase in serum cortisol is an appropriate response post-exercise. Horses meeting the subjective criteria for overtraining have a reduced cortisol response to a standardized exercise test that occurs concurrently with a decrement in maximal exercise capacity. ACTH response is normal, as is the response of the pituitary to exogenous releasing hormones. These results indicate that the acquired defect does not involve deficiencies in the pituitary or the adrenal cortex. Rather, the defect appears to be hypothalamic in nature, perhaps in the ability of the hypothalamus to convert the physiological stress of exercise into activation of the hypothalamic/pituitary/adrenal axis. The subsequent steps leading from impaired cortisol release to poor performance are not known, but may be related to other changes associated with overtraining, including weight loss without a decrease in food intake, irritability, and impaired immune function.

Conclusion

The physiological demands of athletic performance are different from basal metabolism, and thus require different capacities of those systems that support exercise. The potential to adapt to those demands is inherent in horses, but the actual adaptations require activity-specific stresses that, when applied carefully, trigger the expression of those adaptations. Furthermore, the absence of continued exercise stress will eventually result in a return to the physiology of basal metabolism. Injury and overtraining are more likely when the application of exercise stress exceeds the capacity of the tissues to respond and adapt. Through a careful understanding of the functional changes required to support exercise, and the mechanisms by which those changes are triggered, horsemen can more effectively manage their equine athletes.

Additional Reading

Rivero JL, Ruz A, Martí-Korff S, Estepa JC, Aguilera-Tejero E, Werkman J, Sobotta M, Lindner A. *Effects of intensity and duration of exercise on muscular responses to training of thoroughbred racehorses.* J Appl Physiol. 2007 May;102(5):1871-82.

Yamano S, Eto D, Kasashima Y, Hiraga A, Sugiura T, Miyata H. *Evaluation of developmental changes in the coexpression of myosin heavy chains and metabolic properties of equine skeletal muscle fibers.* Am J Vet Res. 2005 Mar;66(3):401-5.

Yamano S, Eto D, Sugiura T, Kai M, Hiraga A, Tokuriki M, Miyata H. *Effect of growth and training on muscle adaptation in Thoroughbred horses.* Am J Vet Res. 2002 Oct;63(10):1408-12.

Rivero JL, Talmadge RJ, Edgerton VR. *Correlation between myofibrillar ATPase activity and myosin heavy chain composition in equine skeletal muscle and the influence of training.* Anat Rec. 1996 Oct;246(2):195-207.

Rivero JL, Talmadge RJ, Edgerton VR. *Myosin heavy chain isoforms in adult equine skeletal muscle: an immunohistochemical and electrophoretic study.* Anat Rec. 1996 Oct;246(2):185-94.

Firth EC. *The response of bone, articular cartilage and tendon to exercise in the horse.* J Anat. 2006 Apr;208(4):513-26.

Smith RK, Goodship AE. *The effect of early training and the adaptation and conditioning of skeletal tissues.* Vet Clin North Am Equine Pract. 2008 Apr;24(1):37-51.

Mukai K, Ohmura H, Hiraga A, Eto D, Takahashi T, Asai Y, Jones JH. *Effect of detraining on cardiorespiratory variables in young thoroughbred horses.* Equine Vet J Suppl. 2006 Aug;(36):210-3.

Buhl R, Ersbøll AK, Eriksen L, Koch J. *Changes over time in echocardiographic measurements in young Standardbred racehorses undergoing training and racing and association with racing performance.* J Am Vet Med Assoc. 2005 Jun 1;226(11):1881-7.

Young LE. *Cardiac responses to training in 2-year-old thoroughbreds: an echocardiographic study.* Equine Vet J Suppl. 1999 Jul;30:195-8.

Roberts CA, Marlin DJ, Lekeux P. *The effects of training on ventilation and blood gases in exercising thoroughbreds.* Equine Vet J Suppl. 1999 Jul;30:57-61.

Evans DL, Rose RJ. *Cardiovascular and respiratory responses to submaximal exercise training in the thoroughbred horse.* Pflugers Arch. 1988 Mar;411(3):316-21.

Rivero JL, van Breda E, Rogers CW, Lindner A, van Oldruitenborgh-Oosterbaan MM. *Unexplained underperformance syndrome in sport horses: classification, potential causes and recognition.* Equine Vet J. 2008 Sep;40(6):611-8.

de Graaf-Roelfsema E, Keizer HA, van Breda E, Wijnberg ID, van der Kolk JH. *Hormonal responses to acute exercise, training and overtraining. A review with emphasis on the horse.* Vet Q. 2007 Sep;29(3):82-101.

In: Rehabilitating the Athletic Horse
Editors: H. W. Jann et al., pp. 31-36

ISBN: 978-1-678-1-60876-672-7

Chapter 3

REGIONAL THERAPY

G.E. "Bud" Fackelman
DVM, Dr med vet, DACVS, DECVS,
Oklahoma State University College of Veterinary Medicine,
Center for Veterinary Clinical Sciences, Stillwater, Oklahoma, USA

ABSTRACT

This chapter deals with the special treatment of the injury for which the horse now finds itself in a rehabilitation program. As such, most of the methods described will be used in the early phases of the program, when healing of wounds, both surgical and otherwise inflicted will be of paramount importance. We will deal mainly with physical therapeutic measures and describe their practical applications. The subject of postoperative antibiosis has received ample coverage elsewhere [1], and will not be examined in any depth here. Regional physical therapy is directed at reduction of pain, avoidance of adhesions, and maintenance of a physiologic range of motion.

INTRODUCTION

Understanding the pathophysiology of soft tissue orthopedic injuries is the key to their successful treatment [2]. We will use the superficial flexor tendon (SFT) as an example, but generalizations may be drawn to apply to all other similar tendo-ligamentous structures.

The biomechanics of breakdowns in the equine forelimb have been studied in detail [3], and we are all familiar with the backward-bending fetlock of the lead leg; and, that the limb in question is at that time experiencing forces totaling several times the animal's body weight. With that picture in mind, it is not difficult to imagine that a fiber or two of the superficial flexor tendon may have been stretched beyond their breaking point. If the strain continues and/ or worsens due to overall fatigue, then larger groups of fibers fail, and the entire structure is gradually placed in jeopardy. In most cases, the exertion is not allowed to progress to total failure, and we are faced, sometimes several hours after competition or training, with the slowly enlarging, soft, painful disfigurement known as a "bowed tendon".

Less extensive swellings in the same area that resolve themselves spontaneously have sometimes been termed "warnings".

The root source of this inflammation is the rupture of tiny blood vessels within the tendon that provide nutrition to the cells responsible for metabolism, and, elaboration and repair of the tendon's microstructural elements. These small vessels have been shown to ultimately stem from one major artery that enters the SFT just above the carpus [4]. When this blood supply is interrupted anywhere along its path, the cells that depend upon it die, and these small areas of dead tissue incite a clean-up response that we perceive as inflammation (heat, redness, swelling, pain). Just how dynamic and fragile this metabolic system is may be deduced from recent articles on the relationship of certain antibiotics to tendon rupture [5]. As the natural repair response progresses, the originally linearly arranged (and now dead) tendon fibers are replaced with new wavier ones easily recognized under a microscope. These "newbies" must then be trained into becoming as straight and strong as their predecessors – and therein lies the problem.

It is difficult or impossible for a trainer to know exactly where (s) he is with any given horse, given its external appearance. Ultrasonic imaging holds the best promise for evaluating soft tissue damage/ healing [6], but evaluation must be carried out by skilled personnel, and even then we may fall prey to over-optimism. As mentioned in our chapter on the Overall Philosophy of Rehabilitation, it is far better to err on the side of conservatism here, and continue training for strength and endurance before taking speed up a notch. A mistake at this juncture can set the athlete back to square one, or even be career-ending.

With this very basic understanding of the nature of soft tissue orthopedic injury, we are ready now to consider various therapeutic modalities. Again, we will use the SFT as an example, but the principles involved apply to all other similarly constituted structures.

Range of Motion Exercises

Moving the skeletal elements bridged by an injured soft tissue structure works to prevent motion-limiting scar by "telling" the tissue it needs to elongate/ become more flexible. In the case of the SFT and other fetlock support structures (e. g., deep flexor tendon, inferior check ligament, suspensory ligament), this means moving the fetlock and digital joints through whatever range of motion that is non-painful. When the injury is acute, this range will be very limited, and should not be forced. In the acute stage, it may be helpful to apply ice or cold water hosing to reduce discomfort before exercise is initiated. If this is still too painful, ethyl chloride spray [7] may be applied for the so-called "spray and stretch technique", also used in humans – especially children – for passive manipulation of a painful extremity. At first, the limb is moved passively, and then the animal is asked to initiate the movement itself – as in having it present its hoof for cleansing. This voluntary effort activates the "muscle pump", a great aid in moving lymph containing products of inflammation proximally, thereby reducing edema.

Hot – Cold Therapy

About three days later, alternating applications of heat (simple bandaging, warm water DMSO) and cold (hosing, ice massage) further reduce swelling. The reduction in edema by this alternating hot-cold therapy is thought to occur via the opening of greater numbers of peripheral lympho-venous anastomoses, known to occur in humans, and shown to also be present in the limbs of horses [8].

As local swelling and pain begin to subside, ROM exercises can take place over a greater range, and for a greater number of repetitions. However, the therapist must keep the manipulations below the threshold of pain. This is especially important if articular disease is the major problem, or even just a contributing factor (see also Chapter 8). When the limb may be moved painlessly through a full range of motion with little or no resistance from the patient, an Exercise Prescription may be developed, an example of which is given under Controlled Exercise Programs below.

Ultrasound

As opposed to diagnostic ultrasound, used to monitor the progress of healing of soft tissue orthopedic lesions, therapeutic ultrasound [9] may used to help resolve muscle spasm and thereby act in an anti-inflammatory, analgesic way. The operator must be skilled in the identification of spastic areas or trigger points, and accurately apply the sonic energy to "loosen" the tissues and relieve the pain. This usually requires a number of treatments spread over several weeks, but the relief can be long lasting and even permanent. The wise trainer will seek out these lesions, which may be either the animal's primary problem, or a secondary one at some distance from the main lesion.

Post-Surgical Therapy

All of the above applies as well to animals that have had surgery, with the added consideration of protecting the operative wound. The latter must be covered by an occlusive dressing when necessary (e. g., during hydrotherapy), and redressed following each session. In addition, the surgeon may have special orders regarding antibiotic and analgesic medications. Communications between the surgical team and postoperative care personnel must remain open, and any questions or complications must be made known to all parties concerned - immediately. It is most important that expectations regarding healing are well-known to all personnel, and that benchmarks (e. g., cessation of drainage, suture removal, etc.) are set in advance, and recorded as they are reached. In fracture patients, a schedule for postoperative radiographic evaluations should be set and strictly followed. Similarly, if external fixation has been applied, the time for its removal or renewal must be known to all.

Exercise Prescriptions

When the horse is ready to be turned over to the owner/ trainer for care (see Chapter 1), it should be accompanied by a clear set of instructions regarding both local and general rehabilitation. The former should include information on the various entities mentioned above, and a carefully planned exercise regime.

An example of such a set of instructions is:

Exercise Prescription - Standard

- Rest, passive manipulation 2wks - soft tissue healing
- Hand walk 2wks
- Ride/ Drive
- 30 min W 2x/ day 4 wks
- 20 min W - 5 min T - 20 min W 2 wks *
- 15 min W - 10 min T - 15 min T 2X/ day - 2 wks
- 15 min W - 15 min T - 15 min W 2X/ day - 2 wks
- Passive ROM exercises below pain threshold
- Daily throughout

- Navicular Desmotomy
- Rest - 2 wks
- Hand walk - 1 wk
- Ride/ Drive
- 20 min W - 5 min T - 20 min W - 1 wk
- 15 min W - 10 min T - 15 min W - 2X/ day 1 wk*
- 15 min W - 15 min T - 15 min W - 2X/ day - 1 wk
- Medications
- NSAID's - 1 wk
- Vasoactive agents - 6W on/ 6W off

- Sesamoiditis
- Standard Exercise Prescription
- Medications
- Vasoactive agents
- Intraarticular Na hyaluronate

- Spavin
- Standard Exercise Prescription
- May need to lengthen initial phase
- May need to "back down" from 3rd to 2nd stage, then repeat

- Stress Fractures
- Osteostixis
- Standard Exercise Prescription +
- Following fourth stage, add 5 minutes gallop

- Increase every 2 weeks until maximum speed @ 20 wks
- Tendinitis
- Standard Exercise Prescription*
- Medications
- NSAIDs - 1 wk
- Local DMSO alternating with cold water

- Tendovaginitis
- Standard Exercise Prescription*
- Medications
- NSAIDs - 1 wk
- Intrathecal Na hyaluronate
- Local DMSO alternating with ice packs

- Carpal Tunnel Syndrome (CTS)
- Study anatomy carefully
- Practice on cadaver specimens!
- CTS – Aftercare
- As for tendovaginitis
- Inject HA @ drain removal (ca. 48 hrs) & @ 6 wks
- Lengthen phase 2 in Std Exercise Prescription work for accessory carpal fracture

- Dorsal Spinous Process Removal
- Standard Exercise Prescription
- Insert Treadmill/ Swim training between phase 2 & 3
- Evaluation/ Massage of Longissimus mm.
- Medications
- Muscle relaxants
- Trigger point injections

The above program attempts to simplify communications by establishing a basic, core set of interventions that are then augmented or modified according to the specific local lesion. The recommendations have been developed over a period of years, and still need “tweaking” according to an individual animal’s response, and individual clinician’s preferences. You will note that we recommend riding or driving early in the program, if the horse’s progress permits. We feel that the added weight or strain is insignificant in an animal already trained to saddle and/ or harness, and that the rider/ driver is likely to have a great deal more control over the animal in that position. The program is presented here only as a suggestion, and should provide a good place to start, if a program is not yet in place at your facility. When developing your own program, it should be at least as specific as the one above, and tailored to the interventions common at your own center.

CONCLUSION

Regional therapy for orthopedic injuries is directed at the reduction of edematous swelling, inflammation and pain. In conjunction with systemic anti-inflammatory agents and analgesics, modalities such as range-of-motion exercises (with our without cryotherapy depending on degree of discomfort), hot-cold therapy, and therapeutic ultrasound may be used to achieve these ends. When the patient no longer experiences motion limiting pain at the site of an injury, a carefully escalating exercise program may be instituted. If, at any stage in the program, pain should return, then the therapist must retreat to a previous level of less intense exercise, and progress more slowly until discomfort disappears.

REFERENCES

[1] Orsini JA. *Surgical wound infection and antibiotic prophylaxis. In: Auer JA, editor.* Equine Surgery: WB Sanders Co.; 1992; 38-91.

[2] Fackelman GE. *The nature of tendon damage and its repair.* Equine Vet J, 1973 Oct;5(4):141-9.

[3] Rooney JR. *Biomechanics of lameness in horses*. Baltimore: Williams & Wilkins Co.; 1969.

[4] Kraus-Hansen AE, Fackelman GE, Becker C, Williams RM, Pipers FS. *Preliminary studies on the vascular anatomy of the equine superficial digital flexor tendon*. Equine Vet J, 1992 Jan;24(1):46-51.

[5] Szarfman A, Chen M, Blum MD. *More on fluoroquinolone antibiotics and tendon rupture*. N Engl J Med, 1995 Jan 19;332(3):193.

[6] Gillis CL. *Rehabilitation of tendon and ligament injuries*. Proc Amer Assoc Eq Pract, 1997:306-9.

[7] Kraus H. *Diagnosis and treatment of muscle pain*. Chicago: Quintessence Pub. Co.; 1988; 14-15.

[8] Fackelman GE, Auer J, Wirth W. *Lymphography in the horse*. Vet Med Small Anim Clin, 1974 May;69(5):614-28.

[9] Speed CA. *Therapeutic ultrasound in soft tissue lesions*. Rheumatology (Oxford), 2001 Dec;40(12):1331-6.

In: Rehabilitating the Athletic Horse
Editors: H. W. Jann et al., pp. 37-65
ISBN: 978-1-678-1-60876-672-7

Chapter 4

STEM CELL THERAPY. SHOCK WAVE THERAPY

Scott Reiners
DVM, Diplomate ACVS,
Mountain View Equine Hospital, Virginia, USA

ABSTRACT

This chapter is an overview of two controversial therapies: stem cell and shockwave. The chapter begins by giving the reader a brief overview on the effects stem cells have on cells and the surrounding tissues. The author then explains the different types of stem cell therapies used in the horse and how they are collected and cultured. The stem cell section is concluded with case studies to describe how the author has used stem cells. The chapter flows into a brief description on how shockwaves are formed and transmitted. The chapter concludes with usage of the shockwave therapy for different conditions in the horse.

INTRODUCTION

With the advancement of medicine and a higher caliber of equine athlete on the show circuit, a need has risen to get the athlete back to work at a faster rate. For some horses, time off is lost income for both the trainer and owner. Veterinarians are feeling the pressure to deliver treatments which will quickly return athletes to soundness along with high success rates. This pressure has led to the development of novel therapies and controversial treatments including stem cell therapy and extracorporeal shock wave therapy. By no means do these therapies replace traditional treatments or surgical intervention, but in many cases they are used supplementary and synergistically.

Stem Cells

What are Stem Cells?

To understand how to incorporate stem cell therapy, one must first understand the different classifications of stem cells, and how they expedite healing.

For a cell to be a classified as a stem cell, it has to have the ability to differentiate into one or more cell types and propagate in vivo. Potency of the stem cell is defined by its ability to differentiate. Potency is classified as unipotent, multipotent, pluripotent, or totipotent. Unipotent cells differentiate into one tissue cell type, and some do not classify this type as a true stem cell (Figure 1). Unipotent cells reside in tissue, and are responsible for maintenance of that tissue. These cells are host cells, or residing stem cells, which have been influenced to differentiate the tissue around it. For example, as skin wound heals, it is well known that epithelial cells along with fibroblasts, myofibroblasts, etc. will move to the wound margins as healing progresses. The multipotent cell can differentiate or give rise to a number of different cells or tissues. Multipotent cells are defined as having the capability of developing into cells of two different germ layers. The most notable of these is the mesenchymal stem cell, which has the capacity to differentiate into numerous connective tissue and cell types. Multipotent cells have been isolated from many types of mesenchymal tissues in adult mammals, including hepatic [1], neural [2] hematopoietic [3], synovial membrane [4], fat [5], skeletal muscle [6] tissues and the umbilical cord [7,8].

Pluripotent cells can develop across all three germ layers and could develop in theory into a whole organism. The blastula or blastocyst is a pluripotent cell. This definition has been mostly used for embryonic stem cells, but with more recent research, the mesenchymal stem cell can also fit this classification [9]. The totipotent cell is capable of developing into any cell in the body including embryonic tissue and fetal tissue. This classification is designated to the zygote and early embryonic stage cells. Some research has suggested that the cells on the periphery of the blastocyst, trophoblast cells, may also be able to fit this classification [10].

The phenotypic characterization of mesenchymal stem cells (MSC) has been defined in human literature by the Mesenchymal and Tissue Stem Cell Committee of the International Society for Cellular Therapy with the following four minimum criteria:

- MSC when maintained in culture conditions have to adhere to plastic (plastic-adherence)
- MSC must have adipogenic, osteogenic and chondrogenic differentiation ability.
- MSC must express CD73, CD90 and CD105.
- MSC must have negative cellular markers and genes for CD11b, CD14, CD19, CD34, CD45, CD79α, HLA-DR (human leukocyte antigen) and c-kit which are hematopoietic lineage markers [31].

The exact markers of MSC for the horse have not been classified to the best of my knowledge.

Previously tissue healing has been defined in the following stages: the inflammatory stage, the repair stage (subdivided into the fibroblastic phase, the epithelialization phase, and the contraction phase) and lastly the remodeling phase. The fibroblastic phase is the stage when fibroblast migration along a fibrin scaffold occurs. This phase is controlled by growth factors, mainly platelet derived growth factor. It has been determined “higher animals” only have a limited ability to regenerate, therefore, the void remaining after regeneration has occurred, has to be replaced by fibroblast activity, resulting in scarring. We now know most tissue may be regenerated through MSC, however, the quality of regeneration may depend on the cellular environment and the available quantity of MSC. It is now known neural, brain and cardiac tissue, once thought to have no regenerative capabilities, can regenerate with the presence of MSC.

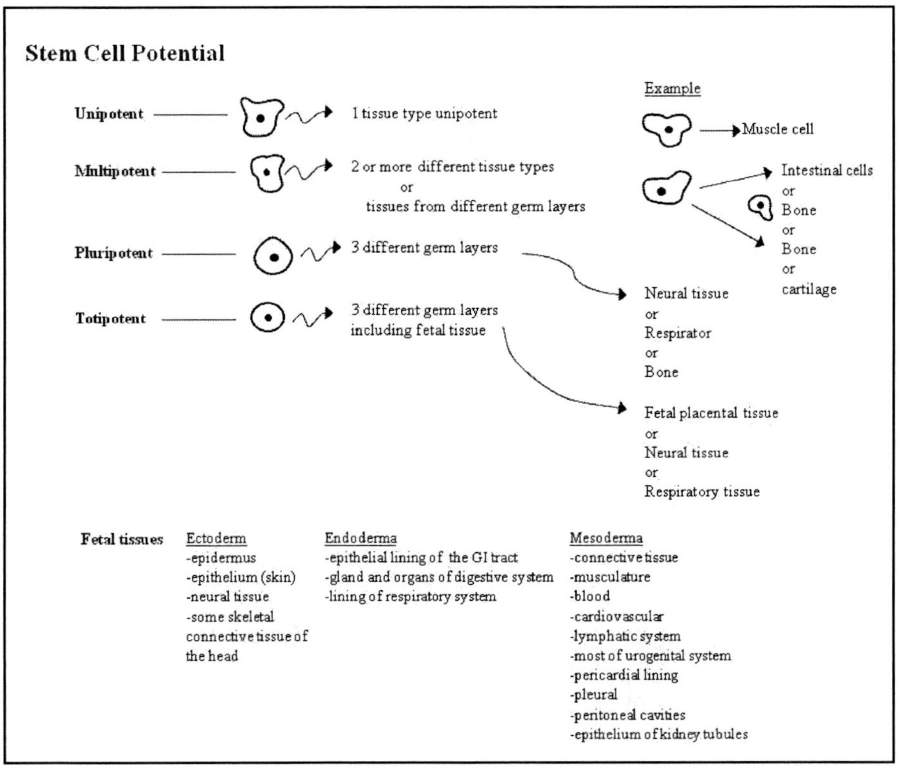

Figure 1. Unipotent cells differentiate into one tissue cell type, and some do not classify this type as a true stem cell.

MSC in vivo can be found circulating within the tissue. An example of a circulating MSC includes hematopoietic stem cells from bone marrow. During repair, MSC are recruited to the site of injury in a process called homing. After arrival to the area, MSC invade and incorporate into normal and abnormal tissue during a process called engraftment. The environment of the tissue in which the stem cells engraft is called the niche. The niche controls the development and differentiation of the stem cell by contact with host cells, growth factors including interleukins, and oxygen content. Research has demonstrated this process when a surgically created lesion in the superficial digital flexor tendon of a horse was injected with labeled MSC. The study demonstrated labeled MSC in the lesion and surrounding healthy tissue. The labeled MSC which had engrafted into the tendon lesion demonstrated tenocyte morphology [11].

The MSC not only engraft into an area, they also secrete potent growth factors. Adipose-derived stem cells secrete vascular endothelial growth factor (VEGF), hepatocyte growth factor (HGF), and insulin-like growth factor 1 (IGF-1) [12]. These factors along with placental growth factor, FGF-2, TGF-β and angiopoietin-1 are known to be considerably proangiogenic [13, 14, 15, 16]. MSC exposure to hypoxia, fibroblast growth, epidermal growth factor, tumor necrosis factor-α can increase the secretion of VEGF, HGF, and IGF-1 [15, 17, 18] (paracrine and autocrine bioactive factors) have a profound effect on surrounding cellular function.

MSC are said to have trophic effects on cells in their vicinity, meaning the molecules secreted can either directly effect cells by intercellular signaling or indirectly effect cells by causing other cells to secrete the active agent. This indirect effect is trophic. The trophic effects are one of the key mechanisms of stem cells causing the up regulation of the surrounding host cells, inhibiting scar formation, inhibiting apoptosis, increasing angiogenesis, stimulating intrinsic progenitor cells to regenerate host tissue and pathways [19].

A study using the caprine stifle joint as a model of osteoarthritis was created by excision of the medial meniscus and transection of the anterior cruciate ligament. After six weeks, the joint was treated with 10 million cells, and the MSC had developed a functional neomeniscal tissue. Articular cartilage degeneration, osteophytic remodeling and subchondral sclerosis were also reduced in the MSC treated joints compared to the controls. The anterior cruciate ligament did not regenerate [20]. This study does not support the trophic theory since the meniscus was removed yet still regenerated. Therefore the question remains: How were MSC able to affect the host tissue cells? Maybe the trophic theory is only partially correct. This study does however demonstrate the homing and differentiation capability of MSC. The homing capability may be controlled by stem cell factor (SCF) which binds to c-Kit. SCF can be found in fibroblasts and endothelial cells. SCF has also been shown to control the melanoblasts' migration from the neural crest to the epidermis, and the primordial germ cells and primordial oocytes migration into the proper position in the body. Here, these cell types possibly play a role in hematopoiesis. Recently, it was found that epidermal growth factor like domain 7 (EGFL7) inhibits notch 1 signaling. Notch signaling plays a role in the formation of astrocytes from neural stem cells, and impedes the formation of neurons and the development of oligodendrocytes. EGFL7 is an antagonist to notch signaling which will allow the neural stem cells to differentiate into neurons, and also plays a role in blood vessel development [21]. Mesenchymal stem cells can differentiate into various cell lines including ectogenic, endogenic and mesogenic, therefore, including everything from skin to neural tissue plus other numerous tissues in between. The exact mechanism is not known yet, but it may involve the Wnt pathway. Wnt, a class of secreted morphogenic ligands, are important in establishing a pattern of development in multicellular organisms. The Wnt pathway involves Wnt proteins binding to surface receptors of cells, mainly frizzled family receptors, thereby causing activation of disheveled family proteins, and changing the amount of β-catenin which interacts with the cell's nucleus. The Wnt pathway has been shown to induce murine embryonic stem cells into mesoderm and endoderm potent cells with a high potential for bone and cartilage differentiation [22]. In a human embryonic stem cell study, Wnt signaling induced hematoendothelial cell development, and Wnt3 influenced more mesogenic committed cells with hematopoietic destiny [23]. Wnt 1 stimulation was associated with nervous system cell regeneration. This is just a short view of the pathway to cellular mutation and/or differentiation.

MSC have immunosuppressive properties in vitro and in vivo, therefore they are said to have a tolerogenic effect on graft acceptance. This effect has been under extensive study in human medical research. In a murine model, a heart was transplanted from the donor to the recipient abdominal region and attached to the aorta. The mice which received donor or recipient MSC prior to the transplant did not reject the transplant, and the mice which received MSC prior to the transplant had a high acceptance rate. Those which received MSC post transplant had a low acceptance rate. Those which received no MSC did not accept the graft. Immunosuppressive properties were said to be associated with the expansion of CD4, CD25, Foxp3, and regulatory T cells [24]. Immunosuppressive properties were optimized in this study when MSC were given via the portal vein causing engraftment of the MSC to the liver possibly interacting with the sinusoidal endothelial cells or the sinusoidal macrophages.

MSC have also been reported to regulate immunosuppression by soluble factors including hepatocyte growth factor and transforming growth factor-β, activated by T cells [24]. MSC have been reported to inhibit B cell proliferation and differentiation [25]. MSC can secrete soluble growth factors such as IL-1β and interferon γ [26]. MSC can initiate apoptosis of activated T lymphocytes via indoleomine 2, 3 – dioxygenase (IDO). MSC expresses IDO, and in the presence of Interferon γ, tryptophan is changed to kynurenine. Tryptophan is needed by lymphocytes to proliferate. MSC also possess inducible nitric oxide synthase which inhibits T cell proliferation via stat-5 phosphorylation. MSC have been shown to express both Cox-1 and Cox-2 which influences synthesis of PGE2, and plays a role in the proliferation of T cells [27,28]. MSC depress phenotype maturation of dentritic cells thus decreasing the capacity for it to stimulate lymphocyte proliferation and decreasing interferon γ, tumor necrosis factor α, and interleukin-2. An in vitro study using dendritic cells derived from monocytes or CD34 cells showed MSC inhibited the up-regulation of CD1a, CD40, CD80, CD86 and human leukocyte antigens-DR (HLA-DR) complex, and prevented up-regulation during dendritic cell differentiation. MSC stopped the up-regulation of CD40, CD86 and CD83 and reduced IL-12 during the maturation process of dendritic cells cultures [29]. The DR complexes are cell surface receptors found in human cell lines. These complexes are involved in regulating T helper cells which then bind to antigens on the B-cells stimulating B-cell proliferation [29].

The HLA-DR has been associated with many diseases including rheumatoid arthritis, Crohn's disease, heart disease, hepatitis, sarcoidosis, narcolepsy, and uveitis. MSC could help to regulate many immune related problems in the horse. Intravenous infusion of MSC has decreased production of Interferon γ (IFN-γ) and tumor necrosis factor [30]. IFN-γ is released by antigen-stimulated T helper lymphocytes which are involved in immune responses. IFN-γ binds to a cell surface receptor protein inducing gene expression, thus producing an antiviral state 1 making the cell less susceptible to infection by the virus. It does this by by inducing phosphorylation of Stat1α protein, enabling it to stimulate transcription, therefor in a viral infection it may block the body's ability to respond to the infection.

It could possibly be used to regulate the destructive events in a mass immune response. Tumor necrosis factor (TNF- α) is a cytokine involved in systemic inflammation and it can stimulate the acute phase reaction. TNF-α is produced mainly by macrophages, but it is also produced by many other cells. Large amounts are released in response to interleukin-1, lipopolysaccharide and other bacterial products. TNF- α can cause problems in the hypothalamus, in the liver, increasing insulin resistance. High concentrations can cause shock-like symptoms, cachexia, a apoptotisis, and up regulate collagenase. With a horse, MSC may be useful for endotoxemic events, cachexia, enteritis, arthritis and insulin resistance syndrome, but further evaluation needs to be done. Increased owner compliance will be needed before all of the uses of MSC can be discovered. In summary, MSC have an immunosuppressive property whether given locally or intravenously. MSC are triggered by inflammatory factors then release soluble factors which will down regulate the immune response. MSC are dose dependant, and also have strong angiogenic factors triggered by inflammation and hypoxic areas which could be useful in ischemic necrosis and post colic surgery.

Stem cells can be obtained from embryonic, fetal, neonatal and adult tissue. Embryonic stem cells are isolated most commonly from the blastocyst. Neonatal or fetal stem cells are commonly isolated from the umbilical cord blood which can be harvested in humans via transcutaneous aspiration of the umbilical cord or from the full term neonate's umbilical cord. Adult stem cells can be isolated in just about all types of tissue, but most commonly taken from bone marrow or adipose tissue. In horses, the most commonly used stem cells are the adult stem cells. Most of the stem cell information is extrapolated rat or human research.

Embryonic Stem Cells

Embryonic stem cells are derived from the inner cell mass of preimplantation blastocysts [10]. The Blastocyst is harvested, and the embryonic disk or the inner cell mass is cultured on feeder-layer cells with bovine serum. Feeder-layer cells can be mouse embryonic fibroblasts, human fetal muscle and skin, human adult fallopian tube epithelium, human foreskin fibroblasts, human adult marrow stromal cells, uterine endometrial cells or human placenta fibroblasts. The feeder cell layer provides a suitable attachment media and soluble factors for undifferentiated human embryonic cell maintenance [33].

Overall, embryonic stem cells are not used extensively because of the difficulty in producing cells other than in research for stem cell therapy in horses. In humans, embryonic stem cell therapy is still in the experimental stages, and has been met with many pit falls. There are ethical considerations in using embryonic stem cells, and teratoma development has been reported after injection. The teratomas have consisted of all three germ layers, so the embryonic stem cell is truly a pluripotent cell. There is a high telomerase expression which is highly correlated with immortality in the human cell lines, thus cell lines can differentiate indefinitely. There is more research and development required before embryonic stem cells can be utilitized on a clinical basis.

Neonatal Stem Cells

MSC are derived from the blood of the umbilical cord after birth, or fromWharton's jelly in both humans and horses. There are conflicting reports in human literature on the potency and availability of MSC derived from the full term neonatal umbilical cord blood (UCB). MSC were unable to be cultured from the UCB because the presence of isolated colony forming units of fibroblastoid cells rather then colony forming units of fibroblastoid adherent cells. MSC-UBC did not differentiate toward the adipogenic lineage compared to adult stem cells likely because the blood is more fetal in origin, and adipose tissue is more adult [34]. UBC is more hematopoietic than mesenchymal. The isolation method for the UCB uses blood which is collected into citrate phosphate dextrose buffer, then diluted with EDTA-phosphate buffer solution. It is then centrifuged and seeded onto a fetal calf serum precoated culture plate and incubated for 12 to 18 hours. Next, the nonadherent cells are removed then cultured for three days, and then cultivated in a 37°C humidified atmosphere of 5% CO2. The expansion medium is then added, which is mesenchymal stem cell growth medium or Dulbecco's modified Eagle's medium-low glucose. When cell colonies reach subconfluence, they are harvested with trypsin or dispase and then washed and replaced. Expansion has been reported to be slower than bone marrow and adipose derived cells. When isolating from the cellular matrix, there is a further process of adding collagenase and washing before seeded can take place.

Adult Stem Cells

Mesenchymal stem cells in the adult can be taken from many different tissues, but the most common are bone marrow and adipose tissue. In humans, obtaining stem cells from bone marrow is a less attractive means of obtaining cells than from fat. In humans, fat is readily available through liposuction with little pain involved and low cosmetic deformation, and is typically readily available and renewable. Harvesting cells from bone marrow is a very painful procedure in humans, and is not always easily accomplished with horses. Bone marrow can be obtained from the tuber coxae or the manubrium through stab incisions with a local anesthetic. The fat is usually removed from the rump near the tail head area with local anesthetic, via a five to eight cm incision. The fat is then dissected from an area where a dimple may remain for an unkown period of time. There has been some liposuction use in horses, which would make the cosmetic appearance for a show horse more appealing. Fat can be obtained from anywhere in the body. Some very fit horses have very little external fat to be found, and an ultrasound examination is needed to find the best area to remove fat. I have always found fat in the furrow between the superficial gluteal muscle and the biceps femoris muscle. Even a small amount of fat (5g) has yielded five to ten million islolated cells, so fit horses seem to have more Stromal-vascular cell fraction per gram of fat than does the obese horse. Stromal-vascular cell fractions are the cells obtained immediately after collagenase digestion of the fat samples.

MSC isolated from bone marrow are labeled as BM-MSC. BM-MSC or hematopoietic stem cells (HSC), when in the marrow, are found along with hematopoietic progenitor cells around or adhered to stromal cells (fibroblasts and osteoblasts) this is call a niche. The hematopoietic stem cells remain in the niche by adhering to extracellular matrix proteins and stromal cells. Stem Cell Factor (SCF) is thought to control the placement of these cells. Some HSC leave the bone marrow and circulate through the body, but then will return to the niche if not used. This relocation is possibly controlled by SCF and chemokine SDF-1. Fetal HSC have a higher sensitivity to SCF than do adult HSC.

After the horse is prepped for either a tuber coxa or manubrium bone marrow biopsy, a needle is used to aspirate bone marrow into a 30ml syringes containing 5ml heparin (1000 IU/ml) diluted with phosphate buffered saline (PBS). 30 milliliters of bone marrow is diluted with 15ml of PBS and centrifuged at 300g for 15 minutes. The supernatant is removed and the pellet is resuspended in PBS and centrifuged again. The cells in the pellet (at the bottom of a conical tube) are resuspended in 12 ml of Dulbecco's modified Eagle medium-low glucose (DMEM/lg) with 10 % fetal bovine serum, 300μg of L-glutamine/ml, 1mmol sodium pyruvate/ml and usually antibiotics. Antibiotocs include sodium penicillin and streptomycin sulfate (100u and 100μg/ml respectively). The suspension is placed in a flask and left in an incubator at 37°C at 90% humidity and 5% carbon dioxide atmosphere for five days. This will give the cells time to attach to the polystyrene surface of the flask. The media is replaced with fresh medium until cells reach subconfluency. The monolayers of MSC are then treated with trypsin then washed again with (DMEM), and replated. This medium is sometimes supplemented with triggering factors to change the commitment of the cells. At this time, I am aware of one laboratory – VetCell, Bioscience Limited, London, United Kingdom - which is processing bone marrow commercially.

MSC are isolated from fat taken by lipoaspiration or resection, and will be all adult stem cells. If resection occurs, the fat pad must be microdissected and washed with PBS. The fat is then digested in .075% cikkagebase type 1 for 30-60 minutes at 37°C with slight agitation. The collagenase is then neutralized with DMEM-lg containing 10% fetal bovine serum. The fatty solution is then centrifuged at 1200g for 10 minutes, and then resuspended with DMEM/lg and filtered through a 100μm nylon mesh. The solution is then centrifuged, decanted and the supernatant is recentrifuged. The erythrocytes are removed from the pellet with erythrocyte lysis buffer and washed in PBS. This end product for this process is the stromal vascular fraction (SVF). The SVF can then either be plated, cultivated, and cultured or it can be sent for use as an injection for horses, dogs or cats. The turn around time is 48 hours, including shipping.–(Vet Stem, Poway, California)

Bone marrow-mesenchymal stem cells (BM-MSC) and adult stem cells (ASC) are presently the most commonly used stem cell lines in horses, dogs and cats. The most noticeable difference between them is the turn around time for treatment. The stromal vascular fraction (SVF) can be received in 48 hours, while the BM-MSC takes about three to six weeks. The SVF contains about 43% stem cells, and BM contains about .002% stem cells per cells collected. The human study "Comparative analysis of Mesenchymal Stem Cells from Bone Marrow, Umbilical cord, or Adipose Tissue" found the colony forming unit frequency was highest in the ACS, and lowest in the umbilical cord blood (UCB), but the UCB could be cultured the longest and had the highest capacity for proliferation. The study also measured the ability of the cells to have mesodermal differentiation. The UCB-MSC had the highest percentage for osteogenic differentiation capacity and BM-MSC had the lowest. Both ASC and BM-MSC had high percentage of adipogenic differentiation capacity, but UCB-MSC had none - all had good chondrogenic differentiation capacity. Adipose tissue in this study contained the highest frequency of MSC. In another study, the adipose tissue around the synovium showed a higher chondrogenic differentiation capacity than subcutaneous adipose tissue. Synovial adipose tissue which derived MSC also had a higher proliferation rate and higher cartilage matrix production. Both ASC and BM-MSC have been effective, but I prefer to use the ACS due to the fast turn-around time.

How are Stem Cells Used?

Stem cell therapy, in my opinion, should be started after the inflammatory stage of wound healing which usually is the first 3-10 days. The healing stage takes place at 10 to 50 days. Tendons, after tendon grafting, start to gain strength between 3 to 6 weekss. This is the optimal time to inject stem cells. The problem is we don't see the acute part of the injury because the owners have initiated stall rest, analgesics and other therapies prior to getting an accurate diagnosis. By the time we diagnose and find the lesion, and make an appointment to complete the harvesting procedure, we are usually well into the healing stage. When used for joint therapy post arthroscopy, we wait ten days before we harvest fat for stem cells. We inject at around 14 days postop. This waiting time ensures we are not going to get a joint infection, horses are off antibiotics and the injection is not as painful. If there is a joint infection it would be flushed immediately, and stem cell therapy will be postponed until it is known that there is no more infection via arthrocentesis and cytology. If you inject too soon, there is a possibility that you may flush the cells out along with the infection. Also since there is a tolerogenic property to stem cells, I feel they may inhibit the immunocapability of the joint in the face of infection. MSC can also help reduce inflammation and thereby reduce pain in osteoarthritis possibly due to their immunosuppressive and chondrogenic capabilities.

Even if soft tissue injuries and joint injuries have been chronic for two months to four years, stem cells can still be used. We have had several cases of chronic deep digital flexor tendon injuries in the navicular bursa and tendon sheath region. We have injected these with good to excellent results. Similar results have been obtained for proximal suspensory injuries. Other lesions including chronic desmopathies of the distal sesamoidean ligaments, collateral ligaments of the distal interphangeal joint and metacarpal/metatarsophangeal joint, and meniscal tears have also been treated with good results.

Joint lesions such as denuded cartilage and osteoarthritis appear to respond well to stem cell therapy. The use of either BM-MSC or ASC does not appear to make a difference in the outcome. MSC have the potential for cartilage and bone repair, and various factors including bone morphogenetic protein (BMP), Hedgehog (Hh), Wnt and Transforming growth can play a role in chondrogenesis. Injecting MSC with hyaluronic acid and polyglycolic acid may help provide viscosity for the joint, but these are probably not needed with MSC. With BM-MSC, we add the hyaluronic acid to the cells, but with the ASC we do not. I have not observed a difference in the cases I have treated.

How to Inject

First, the lesion is confirmed by ultrasound or by MRI except in the cases of spinal cord trauma, in which case the lesions are rarely seen. The normal dose is about 4 million cells for ASCs and 10 million cells for BM-MSC, but this can vary depending on the company producing the cells, the size of the lesion or the joint or area being injected. MSC do respond in a dose dependent manner when using them as immunosuppressants, but to my knowledge there is no set number of cells per area of treatment formulated. In this case you just inject cells, assess response, and if needed, inject again six weeks later. When injecting a lesion, MSC will migrate to other tissue planes as when injecting a tendon lesion. The MSC engraft out to the surrounding tendon crimp and do not stay in the lesion. This is thought to be due to migration, or by the actual insertion of the needle and technique used for injection. During ultrasound guided injections of MSC, the fluid injected can be seen infiltrating surrounding tissue (Figure 2 & 3). When MSC are injected into the joint, some of the MSC infiltrate along the joint surface, but they also engraft to the synovium and likely the cartilage from which the MSC differentiates and can secrete transgenic products and other therapeutic proteins into the joint space. It may be possible to have too many MSC [35]. In a mouse study, genetically modified cells expressed BMP-2, resulting in osteophyte formation and ectopic cartilage formation. In this same study there was an over expression of BMP-2 [36], so it may be possible to inject too many stem cells but I have not found this to be a clinical problem. Large soft tissue lesions may require two injections six weeks apart.

Sterile preparation of the site of injection is of the upmost importance. We use a seven minute scrub with chlorhexidine scrub, then followed with alcohol. It is recommended not to inject antibiotics along with the stem cells because they may alter or damage the cells. In some cases where we feel antibiotics are indicated along with the stem cells, we will either use regional perfusion before injection or inject the joint a half hour before we inject stem cells.

Many times after preparation, we will use a local anesthetic at the site of injection. When injecting the lower limb, we use regional anesthesia. The anesthesia is used so when we guide the needle into the precise location, the horse does not move. Once the needle is in place, it is important the horse does not move when the MSC are being injected. The animal is always sedated when performing this procedure.

Commercial processed BM-MSC and ASCs are transported in a medium, and we will call this transport stem cell suspension. With soft tissue lesions, we use only the content of the syringe sent in order to reduce the volume. With lesions involving large joints, we add hyaluronic acid to the cell mixture prior to loading the syringes. In doing so, we may be damaging some cells so therefore we like to increase the volume going in to the joint.

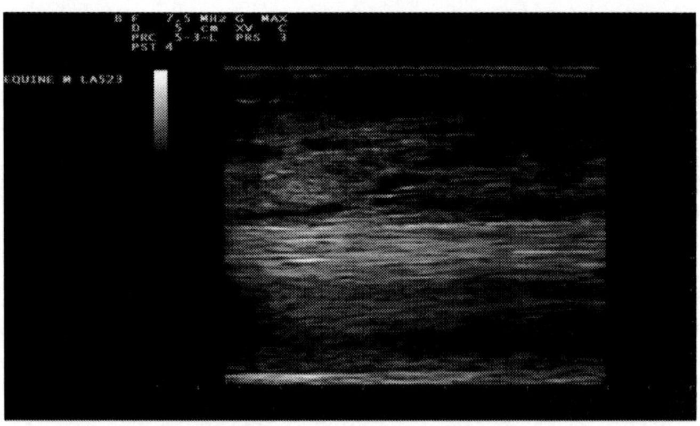

Figure 2. SDFT before injection of stem cell suspension.

We use imaging to guide needle placement. We use both radiograph and ultrasound guided injections. I feel the needle can be placed more precisely with ultrasonic guidance than with radiography. In a diffuse soft tissue lesion, we place multiple needles approximately two to three cm apart. All the needles are placed prior to injection. If fluid flows from the site of the lesion, then it is aspirated prior to injection of stem cells. If injecting into one site and the stem cell suspension appears in the hub of the needle in another site, the stem cell suspension is pushed back into the needle and the needle is removed and then the next site is injected. Diffusion of the stem cell suspension is verified ultrasonographically.

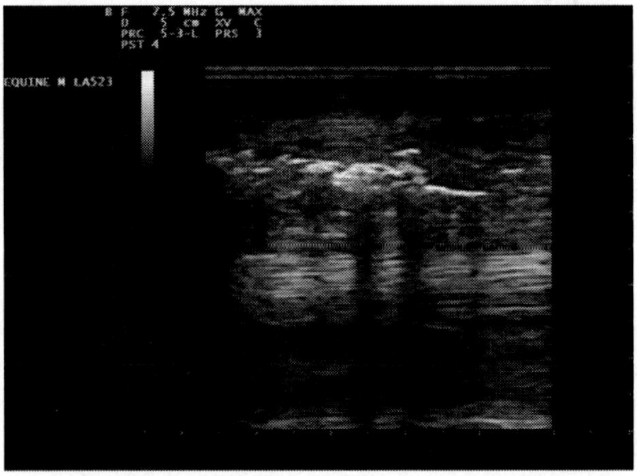

Figure 3. SDFT lesion after injection of stem cell suspension. Note how the suspension diffusely infiltrates the whole lesion and surrounding tissue.

After injection of the stem cell suspension, the area is bandaged or covered with an iodine impregnated impermeable adhesive drape for at least 2 to 24 hours. This time period allows the needle insertion sites to close thus decreasing the chance of any iatrogenic infection. Imaging should be done every three weeks post injection until the lesion is deemed healed. If at six weeks the lesion has not made substantial progress, especially in soft tissue injuries, then more stem cells are ordered. Most commercial processors will have cells banked and frozen. These cells can be replaced and cultivated to make another dose of stem cells. This saves the horse from having another invasive procedure. As of yet, I have not seen a case where more then one reinjection was necessary, but it is possible.

Indications for the use of MSC are not clear at this point. We will use stem cell therapy if the owner can afford it and if it is not contraindicated. I have found no set of criteria for when to use stem cells, but they should not be used in cases of neoplasia, sepsis, marked fracture instability, or between individuals. In cases involving neoplasia, stem cells can differintiate into neoplastic cells. Also, MSC secrete many factors which may enhance the growth or mutation of neoplatic cells. In the presence of sepsis, MSC have immunosuppressive properties and may inhibit the clearing of bacteria. In fracture cases with marked instability, it is possible for the MSC to respond to the stresses placed upon them. Instead of having osteogenic differentiation, there could be a fibroblastic response.

The current recommendation is to place the cells taken from one horse back into the same horse. This is especially important when using ASC because of immunologic reactivity.

It is contraindicated to use shockwave on the area injected for up to 60 days because there is a possibility of injuring or reducing the effectiveness of MSC. If you are going to use shockwave therapy, it may be better to shockwave the area first and then inject the MSC followed by another shockwave at a later time.

It is contraindicated to use corticosteroids with MSC. An in vitro study concluded dexamethasone supplementation may cause BM-MSC to move toward a chondrogenic phenotype, and progress to the formation of bone [37]. This situation to my knowledge has not yet been studied in vivo. Vet Stem has made a recommendation to use one dose of short acting steroids if needed for immediate relief of inflammation, and do not use high doses of antibiotics in the area of injection.

Some of the current uses of stem cell therapy are for osteoarthritis, fracture repair, soft tissue lesions whether chronic or acute, spinal cord trauma, navicular bone cartilage degeneration, longitudinal tears in the deep digital flexor tendon(DDFT), cartilage degeneration in any joint, meniscal tears, desmitis in any ligament whether chronic or acute and tendinitis whether chronic or acute.

Meniscal tears which are seen most often in "cutting horses". These lesions can be career ending injuries for horses, and can also lead to osteoarthritis. Arthroscopy can be performed on some of these tears, and the options are debridement if a small tear or suturing. Some horses do get better with surgery, but many do not. In my opinion, if the lesion lends itself to arthroscopy, then it should be performed and stem cell therapy should be used in conjunction with the surgery. While performing the arthroscopy, the fat around the stifle is an excellent source for stem cell extraction.

Cartilage degeneration in a pastern joint, areas in the fetlock or other difficult to reach places may lend themselves to arthroscopy, but if arthroscopy is not an option, then stem cell therapy should be considered for maintenance of the joint.

Desmitis and tendinitis, whether it is a core lesion or a diffuse thickening of the ligament either chronic or acute, should be candidates for shockwave therapy and stem cell therapy. There are other modalities such as fasciotomies, neurectomies, bone marrow injections, IRAP injections, PRP injections, corticosteroid injections, iodine and almond oil injections, glycosaminoglycan injections, or pin firing. All have had some form of success and failure. I prefer shockwave and stem cell injections if it is within the owner's economic and financial means.

Osteoarthritis of the distal hock joints and pastern joints are difficult to medically treat once the process starts. Treatment of these joints with shockwave and stem cell therapy has lead to favorable results.

Spinal cord trauma that is non-responsive to other treatments, or if the horse continues to stay ataxic after all other modalities have been exhausted, are candidates for stem cell therapy.

Laminitis problems in horses can also be treated with stem cell therapy. If the horse has not improved with standard treatments, stem cell therapy in theory should be the treatment of choice. MSC should reduce the inflammatory response, regulate neovasculization and re-build laminar tissue. More research needs to be done in this area.

Stem cell therapy could also be used for systemic toxicity, insulin resistance, OCD, COPD, uveitis, autoimmune disease and laminitis. As of right now, I have not had the chance to use stem cell therapy for these problems. Stem cell therapy has many uses we have only touched upon as of now. With more people demanding faster and better results, stem cells therapy usage will likely expand.

At present, we have not had a case where stem cells were used that did not improve a lameness score. In many cases, they have returned to complete soundness and continued to work. The following are a few case examples.

Case Example 1

An eight-year-old Quarter Horse gelding, used as a western pleasure show horse, was found down, and unable to stand inside his stall after feeding. The horse was treated initially with DMSO, corticosteroids and NSAIDS. Later that day, the horse was able to rise and stand but unable to walk out of his stall. Treatment continued, and test results for equine protozoal myeloencephalitis, equine herpes and west nile were all negative. The lesion appeared to be localized to the cervical region. Radiographs and ultrasound revealed osteoarthritic changes on articular facets of C4, C5 and C6. On C3, there appeared to be a small fragment. The vertebral canal diameter was normal. The horse's owner declined a myelographic examination and an MRI. The horse continued to improve for the next two to three months, but then his improvement became stagnant. At six months the horse stumbled and could not run without tripping and falling. He was too unstable to ride. We used ASC taken from the adipose tissue from the rump. Only about 27 grams of fat was able to be harvested from this horse - the 27 grams yielded 3.1 million cells according to the commercial lab (Vet Stem). The horse was then placed under general anesthesia in lateral recumbency. The horse was prepped for an AO spinal tap. The spinal needle was placed through the dura mater, cerebrospinal fluid was obtained and then the 10mls of stem cell suspension was injected through a hemo-nate filter. The horse was recovered in a sling and recovery was excellent. The horse was mildly more ataxic for the first 24 hours after the injection. He was treated with one dose of corticosteroids and NSAIDs. Over the next six weeks he improved enough to be ridden. Later that year, he was showing at the same level as he was prior to the ataxic event. The reason for his recovery is unknown. It may be due to the stem cell's ability to cause an immunosuppressive effect within the subarachnoid space. With all the corticosteroids and NSAIDS this horse had been given along with the fact the cerebrospinal fluid was normal, tells me the immunosuppressive response was a small part of the improvement. It is likely there was a defect in the spinal cord or a focal lesion in the dura mater and the stem cells repaired the area. We will never know. There have been four to five other reports using ASCs in epidural space, but none have been written and I am not aware of their outcomes.

I believe ASC are safe to use on central nervous system problems in the horse at this time. More research is absolutely needed to find out what happens to the stem cells once they are in cerebrospinal fluid. I do not know if the BM-MSC have been used for this type of procedure in the horse.

Case Example 2

A four-year-old Quarter Horse gelding used for western pleasure had a left hind high suspensory injury which had been previously treated 10 weeks earlier by another veterinarian. The horse had been stall rested for two months, during which time a right forlimb lameness developed. The right forelimb lameness was localized to the foot, and the left hind limb suspensory ligament was very thick and only mildly sensitive to palpation. MRI of the left hind suspensory ligament revealed a severe, chronic –active desmitis, which originated at the origin, and extended 10cm distally. The cross-sectional area was 4.1cm^2, and there were possible adhesions to Mt4. The right front foot had focal fibrocartilage degeneration of the navicular bone and solar frog and heel hemorrhagic exudates. The front navicular bone was treated with IRAP (interleukin-1 receptor antagonist proteins) and shoeing changes. The left hind limb was treated with ASCs taken from the rump area of the horse. Only 13.2 grams of fat could be removed from the horse but that yielded 5.3 million cells (Vet Stem). Unfortunately, there was only enough for one dose. The horse was then sedated, and a local infusion of mepivacaine was placed in four different areas along the proximal suspensory ligament region. Four separate needles were placed along the proximal suspensory area using ultrasonic guidance. Each area was injected with approximately one million cells. With ultrasound, it was possible to see the stem cell suspension diffuse throughout the lesion. The tarsometatarsal joint was also injected with 40mg of depo medrol, 11 mg hyaluronic acid and 50mg amikacin. The horse was placed on controlled exercise for one month hand walking. During that month, the suspensory ligament reduced to half the size it had been when the horse first arrived. Ultrasound measurements were 2.0c m^2 in the left hind limb proximal suspensory ligament, and the right hind limb measurement was 1.7cm^2. At this time, the horse was sent home to the trainers to continue rehabilitation which consisted of hand walking for 15 to20 minutes three times a day for one month, and then re-ultrasound or MRI to see if he could go back to work. The horse was transported out of state where he was lost to follow up until the owner called three months later to inform us the horse was doing great, and that he would be showing all show season. He showed at the World Quarter Horse Show that year.

This case shows a fit horse, even if he has only a small amount of fat, usually has a fairly dense population of viable cells. The pattern of healing in chronic diffuse lesions is usually similar to this case. The cross sectional area usually decreases over the first four to six weeks. If the cross sectional area of the proximal suspensory ligament had not continued to decrease and the horse stayed consistently lame, then another MRI would be indicated or the adhesion seen on the Mt4 to the suspensory ligament may have to have been transected along with injecting the suspensory ligament again with stem cells. I feel the cross sectional area of the lesion is one important indicator of healing along with parallel fiber alignment and isoechoic to normal tendon or ligament. The ultrasound examination needs to include to opposite limb for comparison. When ultrasounding the proximal suspensory ligament, it is necessary to determine which body of the suspensory is injured. In the front suspensory ligament there is a medial and lateral body, and in the hind limb there is a short branch of the plantar ligament which makes up the superficial part of the suspensory ligament. At the origin the proximal suspensory ligament, there is a lateral, middle and medial body divided by bundles of connective tissue, muscle fiber and fat (as per Dr J-M Denoix). The bodies can be seen with ultrasound by doing a comparison of off set (angling the probe slightly to enhance contrast) and normal ultrasound. In the Quarter Horse, most problems occur in the middle body.

Case Example 3

A 14-year-old Hanoverian gelding was retired from show jumping, and was in dressage training when he came up from the pasture 3/5 lame. The trainer thought it was a possible foot abscess, and the horse was treated as such. On presentation, the horse had no heat in the foot but had swelling up to the fetlock. Hoof tester exam was negative, but was painful at the region of insertion of the superficial digital flexor. The horse was treated with NSAIDs and cold compression therapy. The horse's lameness worsened to a 4/5 lameness. Radiographs showed an osteophyte on the dorsal proximal aspect of P2, and a slightly increased sclerotic appearance to proximal P1. Ultrasonic examination revealed a possible longitudinal tear in the DDFT, and thickening of the lateral distal oblique sesamoidean ligament, effusion of the pastern joint and metacarpophalangeal joint with osteophytosis in various areas along proximal P1. The joint fluid from the coffin joint, fetlock joint and pastern joint was normal.

The coffin joint, digital tendon sheath, pastern joint and fetlock joint were treated with 22mg hyaluronic acid, 4mg triamcinolone and 100mg of amikacin. NSAID were given. Regional perfusion of antibiotics and lidocaine was performed which improved the lameness to a 3/5 for about two days after the treatment. An MRI was performed which revealed P1 bone injury associated with an increase in vascular response to some intramedullary bony insult, pastern joint effusion, desmitis of the lateral and medial distal oblique sesmoidean ligaments, osteoarthritic changes of the metacarpophalangeal and metacarposesmoidean joints (articular cartilage degeneration and subchondral sclerosis in the sagittal ridge of Mc3). The horse was treated with regional perfusion of Tildren. Fat was obtained from the rump and within three days, the fetlock joint, digital tendon sheath, pastern joint and the lateral oblique distal sesamoidean ligament were injected with ASC. During a three-day period the horse became a 1/5 lame. The horse went home with a rehabilitation regime of 15-25 minutes of hand walking two to three times a day, and stall rest for 30 days then free turn out for 45 days, and then light riding after that time. Five months after the severe lameness, the horse was back to training as a show jumper and one year later he was back to grand prix jumping. The owner said he had been retired previously because he could not keep him sound. No further interarticular therapy has been required.

A helpful lesson learned from this case was the MRI should have been done before the first initial treatment, but after the first injections this horse started to improve. The reason for such severe pain may have been the combination of the horse's problems. Infrequently do we find just one problem which needs to be treated in a lameness case. Most of the lameness cases we see have multiple problems We have not been able to re-examine the horse, nor has it had a follow up ultrasound or MRI. The horse was moved to Florida soon after discharge from the hospital. The owner did send us a video of the horse jumping when we called for a follow-up.

Case Example 4

A seven-year-old Quarter Horse/Paint gelding used for trail riding and showing presented with severe effusion in the right femoropatellar joint. The horse had been treated for about a year with chiropractic therapy and other joint therapies. Arthroscopic examination revealedsevere cartilage erosion on the articular surface of the patella. About 2/3 of the patellar cartilage was absent and there was cartilage fibrillation and severe synovial flare through out the joint. The cartilage was curetted, and the joint was treated with IRAP for one year. The horse was intermittently lame for over a year. Radiographs were taken which showed fragmentation of the patellar margins. A subsequent arthroscopic examination revealed multiple fragments along the apex of the patella. The eroded cartilage on the patella was covered with fibrocartilage, and had some fibrillation. The femoral cartilage was cracked and had areas which were lifting off the subchondral bone, and areas of very thin cartilage. The synovium was normal in appearance. The cartilage flaps and the fragments were removed and due to the extent of the cartilage problems, stem cells were elected to be used as a post-op joint treatment. Fat was removed from the rump area. Ten days after surgery, four million cells were injected along with 22 mg of hyaluronic acid. The horse continued to improve and the effusion decreased. At two months, the owner started light riding. After three months following surgery, the horse was brought back for a re-check and was scheduled for another dose of stem cells. The horse was injected with another dose of stem cells and with IRAP.

There was a significant decrease in effusion, and the total protein was <1g/dl. A 1/5 lameness was still evident at this time.

Case Example 5

A 14-year-old American Saddlebred show gelding presented with a 3/5 left forelimb lameness. Ultrasonographic examination revealed a 6mm grade four lesion in the superficial digital flexor tendon, approximately 3-4cm in length. Stem cell therapy was elected and ASCs were injected 10 days after the diagnosis. Physical therapy included three days of stall rest plus hand walking for 15 minutes three times a day. During the horse's re-check at three weeks, the lesion was healing well and the cross sectional area was smaller. Two months after injury, the horse was started under saddle and in three months was sound.The lesion healed very well and the horse is back showing at the same level. Stem cells appear to work well in core tendon lesions (Figure 4, 5, & 6). Some of the diffuse lesions require mor than one injection.

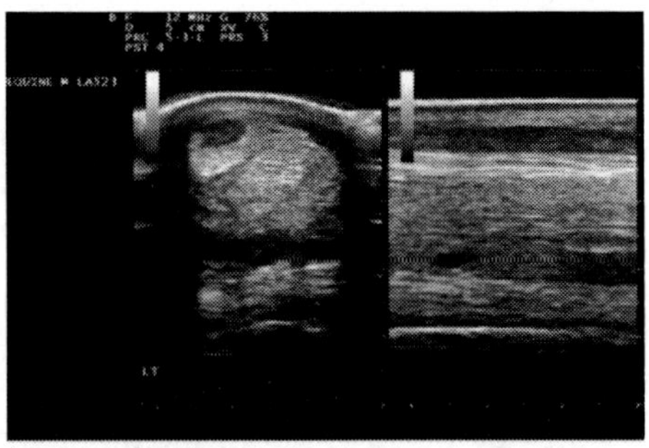

Figure 4. Superficial digital flexor tendon injury.

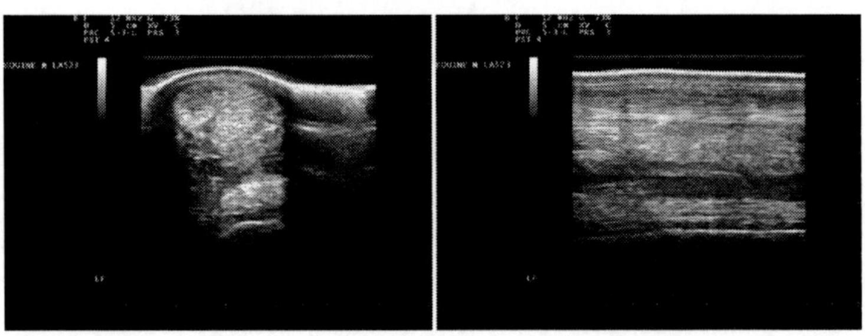

Figure 5. SDFT lesion injected with ASCs on April 8th/27 days after injection.

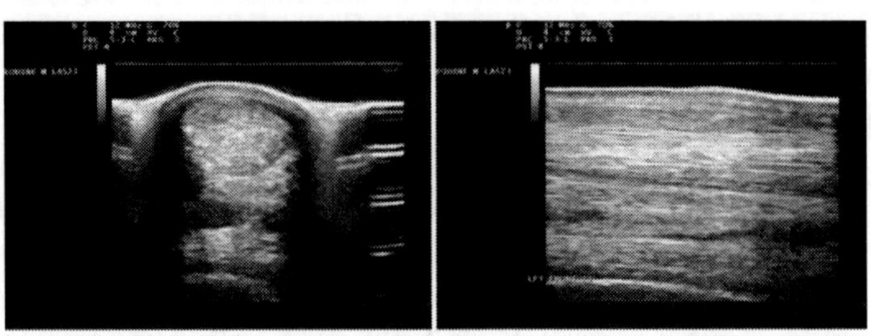

Figure 6. SDFT lesion 48 days after ASCs injection/horse is back into training.

Stem Cell Therapy (Adipose derived stem cell) Proximal Suspensory Desmitis.

	Full work- Upper level	Full work- Lower level	Unresponsive Total	Total
Forelimb	17 (81.0%)	2 (9.5%)	2 (9.5%)	21
Rearlimb	25 (73.5%)	7 (20.6%)	2 (5.9%)	34
Total	42 (76.4%)	9 (16.4%)	4 (7.2%)	55
Acute Injuries	8 (100%)			
Chronic Injuries (> 3 months)	46 (73.9%)			

Upper level – Prior level of work such as performance, hunter, jumper, racing, etc. Lower level – Not to the previous level of work such as smaller jumps or trail horse, etc. Source: Harman; Robert; Orava, J; Cowles B. Vet Stem 12860 Davidson Court, Suite B, Poway, CA 92064. Non-published data compiled from independent veterinarians by authors.

Stem Cell Therapy (Adipose derived stem cell) Flexor Tendon Treatment

	Full work- Upper level	Full work- Lower level	Unresponsive	Total
Forelimb- SDFT	38 (81%)	6 (13%)	3 (6%)	47
DDFT	7 (70%)	2 (20%)	1 (10%)	10
Rearlimb- SDFT	4 (80%)	1 (20%)	0 (0%)	5
DDFT	2 (50%)	2 (50%)	0 (0%)	4
Chronic injuries (> 3 months)	88%			
Acute Injuries	73%			
Severity				
Mild (CSA < 25%)	75%			
Moderate (CSA 26-50%)	83%			
Severe (CSA > 50%)	79%			

(CSA – Cross-Sectional Area) SDFT – Superficial Digital Flexor Tendon DDFT – Deep Digital Flexor Tendon Upper level – Prior level of work such as performance, hunter, jumper, racing, etc Lower level – Not to previous level of work, such as small jumps or trail horse, etc. Project by Vet Stem Inc., Poway, CA

SHOCKWAVE THERAPY

Extracorporeal shock wave therapy (ESWT) was developed in the 1970's for fracturing urinary calculi in humans. As shock wave usage grew in the human field for treatment of calcified tendonitis, plantar fasciitis and insertional desmopathies, we began usage in the horse. In the mid to late 1990's, shockwave was first used in the horse for treatment of proximal suspensory injuries. The treatment spectrum soon grew to include most equine musculoskeletal injuries. As ESWT grew in popularity, research demonstrated the physiologic mechanism for its therapeutic efficacy. Currently, ESWT is a preffered treatment modalitiy for many musculoskeltal problems.

How Shock Waves Work

Shock waves are waves that carry energy. Shock waves, in general, are created by an abrupt discontinuous change in a medium such as air or fluid. They give rise to rapid increase in pressure, temperature and density of flow. As the distance increases, the energy is dissipated. In ESWT the medium we deal with is fluid. Soft tissue is much like a fluid environment hence this is why we can ultrasound soft tissue. There are two types of shock wave modalities used for shock wave therapy; radial and focused. Radial shock wave devices have a focal point of intensity at the skin/device interface and the shock waves disperse it energy in a cone shaped fashion. The focused shock wave has a focal point some distance from the head of the device and the maximum intensity focal point can be delivered at measure depth within the tissues. Focused shock waves are what we will discuss in this section.

There are three main generators of focused shock waves to my knowledge, and they are piezoelectric, electromagnetic and electrohydraulic. The piezoelectric systems use piezoelectric crystals made of ceramic and are seated into a spherical hand piece. These crystals can expand at a high rate of speed when high voltage hits the crystals. The deformation of the crystals in a fluid environment creates a pressure wave in a focused manor. The cone shaped configuration is used to provide a focus for the pressure wave.

The electromagnetic system generates shock waves by the use of two coils which have opposite magnetic fields and a membrane inside a hand piece. When electricity is applied to the coils, a strong magnetic field creates a wave. The electrohydraulic system uses a spark much like a spark plug in a fluid environment. When voltage jumps the gap, it creates a cavitations bubble which expands and then collapses, therefore a wave is formed.

No matter which system is generating the shock wave, they act similarly in that they have a peak pressure at a given distance, and the waves are carried through a fluid environment by the magnitude of the pressure wave. Shock wave energy is described in two ways - peak energy which is the maximum pressure generated, and energy flux density which is basically the amount of energy dispersed in a given area. Energy flux is millijoules per square millimeter (mJ/mm^2).

Shock waves are acoustic waves. Waves are produced when an object moves in a fluid environment, whether it be liquid or gas. When waves are created, molecules are compressed and then molecules compress those next to it and so on. This compression is what forms the wave. The wave is given a focal zone by a large area of wave diverging to a small area. This focal zone is more elliptical in shape. Within this focal zone, there is a variance of pressures from the outside to the inside of the zone. The center has the peak energy. The movement of the compression of molecules is called the acoustic wave. The speed at which it can travel is reliant upon the tissue properties. Acoustic waves travel though water very quickly at about 1500m/s, so hydration of the tissue is important. Compression and tensile acoustic waves create a void or a vacuum. The molecules which have been compressed quickly move to fill in the vacuum, and this process is called rarefaction. The pulse of the wave is roughly 5μs in duration. As soon as a wave is created, it produces an almost instantaneous positive pressure wave of about 30-100MPa. This sudden jump, or transition, is referred to as shock. This transition takes place over a time period of less than 5 ns, then the wave quickly drops to zero in about 1 μs and continues to produce a negative pressure region of about -10MPa for a duration of 3 μs [38].

Velocity of Ultrasound in Various Tissue or Materials.

Material	Velocity (ms^{-1})	Density (kgm^{-1})	Acoustic Impedance ($kgm^{-2}s^{-1}$)
Air	330	1.29	430
Average soft tissue	1300-1800m	1000	1.5×10^6
Bone	3200	1650	5.3×10^6

Acoustic impedance is the product of material density and the velocity of sound traveling through the material. Source: Allisy-Roberts P, Williams JR, Farr RF. Farr's physics for medical imaging. 2nd ed. Edinburgh: New York; 2008; 149.

Shock waves affect density, pressure and particle velocity of the fluid particles. Density is increased because of the compression wave and decreased during the tensile wave; therefore it has a ultrasonic effect. Not only does the acoustic wave move in a linear pattern, but due to the compression, some of the energy is moved into a different direction. This particle velocity could produce stain and cause cell damage. Picture a bunch of people standing in a straight line, then they go and push through a crowd of people. The people that are pushed aside will push the person to the outside of them and then that person will push another person until the person on the outside of the crowd has no one to push, and they jump and move out of the way. Also when the last person in the line gets through, there is a void of people trailing behind him. Since the line has passed, people will start moving into that space. Acoustic wave is the line of people, the tensile acoustic wave is the people moving back to the space, and the particle velocity is the rate and the number of people which are pushed to the outside of the crowd. The rate at which acoustic waves move through the tissue and the density of the material determines it's impedance. Impedance is the ratio of the pressure to the volume displacement. The higher the impedance the faster and more direct the acoustic wave will travel through it. Air, being a very low impedance, will allow very little of the wave to pass therefore abruptly slowing the wave and dispersing the energy to the point of reflection of acoustic wave. When shock waves move through tissue of different impedance, part of the wave will continue to spread or propagate (transmit waves) into new areas, and part of the wave will be reflected back into the original area. So as the shock wave moves through different tissue planes, it loses energy along the way. Each tissue plane will absorb small amounts of energy as the shock wave passes through it therefore the amplitude of the acoustic wave will attenuate as it propagates through tissue.

Besides the mechanical effects on the tissue, there has been some research on the indirect effect of the shock wave. Shock waves cause neovasculization in tissue both in bone and soft tissue. Reports have indicated that proliferating cell nuclear antigen (PCNA), endothelial nitric oxide synthase (eNOS), and vascular endothelial growth factor (VEGF) have been increased with ESWT. Some reports have given this increase of factors as a reason for ESWT stimulated neovasculization. VEGF is in the sub family of platelet-derived growth factors. They are important signaling proteins involved in vasculogenesis and angiogenesis. PCNA is a DNA clamp of sorts. It is important for DNA synthesis and DNA repair. eNOS generates nitric oxide in blood vessels, and is involved with regulating vascular function. These factors may be increased because of inflammation and vascular damage.

In an ESWT in vivo equine research project, osteonal vessels were disrupted and gas pockets were found in the margin of the osteon possibly caused by cavitations. Reddend areas on the bone were found and thought to be caused by the release of hemoglobin from erythrocytes. So the possible reason for neovascularization is the destruction of vessels and cells possibly up regulating the healing events that may have gone dormant [39].

ESWT clinically appears to cause new bone formation, and is used for non-union fractures. In a sheep fracture model, tibial osteotomies were stabilized with external fixators. There were two groups of treated fractures with ESWT and one control [40]. The treated bones had increased endosteal and periosteal new bone formation at the fracture site compared to the control limbs. There are several studies which support the use of ESWT for supplementing fracture repair [41,42]. The reasoning for improvement in new bone growth is unknown, but may lay in the activation of new osteons. In an in vivo study in horses, MC3/MT3 were treated with 2000 pulses at $0.89 mJ/mm^2$. Two limbs were treated with ESWT, one limb was a control, and one limb was treated with periosteal elevation. After 30 days, the ESWT limb had activated osteons throughout the depth of the cortex, and had new formation on the periosteal and endosteal surfaces with less in the cortical bone. On the periosteal elevated limbs, osteogenesis and chondrogenesis was found under the periosteum. ESWT treated limbs had 30% more osteons activated than did the control limb, and 56% more than the periosteal elevated limb. There are conflicting reports on ESWT causing microfractures in bone. An in vivo study failed to demonstrate microfractures [39]. In an in vitro study, microfractures after treatment [43] were found. The in vitro study used frozen and thawed limbs, which in the freezing and thawing process could have lead to ice crystals which can cause the microfractures or the decrease in water content of the bone could had made the bone more susceptible to microfractures.

ESWT clinical has been shown to have an analgesic effect. Pain relief for three to five days has been reported in humans. Clinically, we have used ESWT for osteoarthritic pain in the pastern joint, tarsus and carpus. Most all of the cases have shown improvement by one grade of lameness. Horses with sore feet not related to podotrochleosis have been treated with ESWT, and all of those horses have improved one to two grades of lameness. The reasoning for pain relief is not fully understood currently, but in a rat study, they found that there was degeneration of epidermal nerve fibers in the skin [44]. Other studies have found perineural inflammation, decreased conduction velocities, demyelination and axonal swelling [45].

Shock Wave Treatment Protocols.

Angle of Approach	Probe Depth	Energy Setting	Number of Pulses	Treatment Interval	Indications
Navicular Syndrome					
Through the frog. Through the top of the heel.	20-35mm	* E6 ** 20p *** 0.98 mJ/mm^2	1000 1000 Total: 2000/ treatment	As needed every 6 weeks	Only for Navicular bone degeneration
Sesamoiditis					
Over the body of the sesamoid or directly into lesion of bone.	5mm	* E6 ** 20p	500 per sesamoid	14-20 days 2-3 treatments	Moderate to severe sesamoiditis
Interosseous Ligament Tears Pulled Splints					
Direct through between splint bone and common bone. If chronic with bone formation through the lesion and bony formation.	5-15mm	* E4 ** 15p *** 0.14 mJ/mm^2 * E6 ** 20p	500-750 pulses per site. Do pulse on proximal, distal, & on lesion. Total: 1500 shocks	10 days to 14 days. 2-3 treatments 10 day to 14 days. 3-4 treatments	
Proximal Splint Bone Fractures					
Directly over infected area. Make sure that there is no infection if any curettage and then shock wave.	5-25mm	* E6 ** 20p *** 0.15 mJ/mm^2	*,** 800-1500 pulses *** 600-900 pulses	10-14 days 3 treatments	For non-septic bone fractures
Ringbone and Tarsitis					
Dorsal, medial, lateral over osteophytosis	5-10mm	* E4-E6 ** 15-20p *** 0.15 mJ/mm^2	200 to 300 pulses per area. Total: 800 to 1000 pulses	0 day - 21 days 2-3 treatments	High energy on osteoprolific area. Low energy on rest of joint. Used in conjunction with joint injections.

Shock Wave Treatment Protocols. (Continued)

Angle of Approach	Probe Depth	Energy Setting	Number of Pulses	Treatment Interval	Indications
Stable Stress Fractures					
Over the stress fracture on the fracture line.	Depends on stress fracture. Cannon bone – 5-10mm	* E6 ** 20p *** 0.14 mJ/mm^2	1000-3000 pulses 800 pulses	3-4 weeks	*** 1 week handwalking then treat in 2 weeks. Repeat in 1 week.
Proximal Suspensory Ligament					
Determine the body of the suspensory affected. Medial, lateral, dorsal approach.	Measure depth with u/s. Usually 5-10 medial, lateral. 20-35 dorsal	* E4 to E6 ** 15p to 20p *** 0.15 mJ/mm^2	500 each sight Total: 1500 pulses	10 day to 21 days 3-4 treatments	-Low energy for acute injury -High for chronic injury and insertional disruption.
Distal Suspensory Ligament & Tendonitis					
See ultrasound exam for angles and approaches. Treat complete lesion. Proximal, middle, distal	Measure depth	* E2 - E6 ** 10p - 20p *** 0.09 – 0.15 mJ/mm^2	200-300 pulses/site *** 150 pulses/cm of lesion	3 weeks for 3 treatments	Energy depends if core lesion. Higher with core lesions, lower if more diffuse.
Arthritis					
Cover over full joint.	5mm	* - E6 * - 20p	150 to 200 pulses per area	2-3 weeks as needed	Usually shock wave in 4 regions, try to avoid cartilage
Bone cysts					
Over lesion	5-25mm measure	* E6 ** 20p	1000-2000 pulses	2-4 weeks 3-4 treatments	Use imaging to direct direction of lesion
Sacroiliac					
Left and Right cranial and caudal	35-80mm	* E6 ** 20p	1000 pulses per site	2-3 weeks 2 treatments then as needed	Use imaging to direct direction of approach

Shock Wave Treatment Protocols. (Continued)

Angle of Approach	Probe Depth	Energy Setting	Number of Pulses	Treatment Interval	Indications
Collateral Ligaments					
At insertions and over body of ligament.	Need to measure depth	E4-E6 at insertion. 15-20p. E4-E5 at body of ligament	200-300/site	14-21 days 2-3 treatments	Energy setting depends on chronic or acute.
Muscle Strains, Back Muscle Pain					
Over affected area. Palpate areas of pain or Acupuncture points.	20-35mm 35mm	* E6 ** 20p * E6 ** 20p	150-200 pulses/site 200-300 pulses/site	As needed	
Kissing Spine Lesions					
Over affected area.	Image lesions	* E6 ** 20p *** 0.16 mJ/mm^2	2000-3000 pulses *** 50 pulses/cm length lesion	2-4 weeks 2-5 treatments	

* electrohydrolic unit (Reiners) ** piezoelectric unit (Reiners) *** (McClure S., Weinberger, T. Extracorporeal shock wave therapy: Clinical application and regulation. *Clinical Techniques in Equine Practice* 2003; 2 (4):358-67)

Indications for use of ESWT

The primary use for ESWT is for insertional desmopathies, including both chronic and acute origin and insertional injuries of the proximal suspensory ligament, collateral ligaments of any joint, and nuchal ligament, etc. With desmopathy of the collateral ligament of the distal interphangeal joint, ultrasound first to see if the lesion is visible. If not visible, sometimes you have to lightly rasp the hoof wall to get to the lower insertional area. Use a high setting for about 1200-1500 pulses.

ESWT treatment of any desmopathy or tendinitis has shown benefits and improvement. An equine study using normal tendons and ligaments and ESWT resulted in increased degraded collagen levels acutely, and in six weeks there were decreased collagen levels and an increase in gene expression for COL1 and MMP14. The conclusion was disorganization of the collagen network may be the way ESWT triggers repair of chronic tendinopathies [46]. There is a debate whether to treat acute core injuries, or wait for 10-14 days. I prefer to treat these acute injuries with tendon splitting primarily to remove the blood and serum in the area, and then in 10 days treat with ESWT. Diffuse lesions or thickened tendons or ligaments without core lesions are always treated primarily using low energy settings and 200-400 pulses in several affected areas. I believe this helps reduce the inflammation.

Stress fractures in MC3 and MT3 are commonly treated with ESWT. There is less lay up time in most race horses treated with ESWT than with osteostixis. Training intensity must be reduced after ESWT treatment but strict stall confinement is not required as is the case with osteostixis. Non-union fractures and fracture treatment is as previously stated.

Using ESWT for treatment of pain in laminitis horses is debatable. Theoretically, ESWT may cause more vascular or laminar damage but we have used it on laminitic horses that have had chronic pain. The energy setting is low, and we do multiple areas with low numbers of shocks. We go through the sole, or if the horse is unable to hold the foot up, we have rasped the dorsal hoof and treated the dorsal region of the foot. Some have had pain relief and some have not, but none have worsened after treatment.

Back pain including "kissing spine" lesions appear to respond well to ESWT. The back is radiographed and /or ultrasound to find the lesional area, and the probe is focused on to the lesion. High energy settings with 1500 pulses are used if there is bony proliferation or osteolysis. Treatment of muscle soreness in the back had also shown to respond to ESWT. In these cases, we will palpate for the area of pain and use a moderate to high setting, then start the pulses and watch for muscle fasciculations. If the muscle starts to fasciculate, we will then use about 100-200 pulses in that area. In backs that do not have a primary sore area, we will use the shock wave to stimulate acupuncture points. When stimulating the points, high energy at about 35 mm depth for 200-300 pulses are used. Sacroiliac (SI) joints can be treated with shock waves using ultrasonographic guidance. I have not had exceptional results compared to injections, but I know many veterinarians who have obtained excellent clinical results using this mode of SI treatment. Vertebral articular facet treatment has been conducted with good results. You should radiograph or ultrasound the area to find the articular osteophytosis, and then use the ultrasound to measure and guide placement of the probe. Moderate to high setting is used at 500-1000 pulses. I never shock wave the neck - there are too many important structures to avoid. If ESWT is used in the cervical region, the focal point should not be in a joint or through a joint due to the proximity of the spinal cord. Cavitation and/or spinal cord damage could cause permanent or temporary ataxia or worse.

Practice Tips.

Determine treatment area with imaging.
Measure depth from skin to lesion at every angle of approach.
Do not shock wave through large nerves or vessels.
Do not shock wave through cervical articular facets.
When shock waving the frog on sole of foot, clean and pare away 1mm of brand frog sole should be soaked.
Use ultrasound to determine depth of shock wave.
Use ultrasound to determine best angle of shock wave.
Shock wave will cause inflammation in tissue. Do not shock wave normal tissue if possible.
If probe depth is either too long or too short from the lesion, choose the short probe.
Try to center probe in the lesion.
When possible, use more than one angle of approach.
Never shock wave a possible air filled organ; i.e. Intestine, Lung, Trachea, Esophagus.

Joint pain and arthritis respond very well to ESWT. I have seen a decrease in joint effusion, decreased pain and decreased synovial thickening after treatment. Pain appears to decrease acutely but maintenance treatments are needed for the decrease in synovial thickness and effusion. We use a 5 to 15 mm probe with a moderate energy setting for 500 shocks in three to four areas across the joint. Meniscal tears and subchondral bone cysts have been treated with shock wave. In the few cases I have done by treating the meniscal tears with ESWT, I have seen no healing of the tears, but pain has decreased. Subchondral bone cysts have been treated successfully. Shock waves must be focused on the cyst for successful treatment.

Navicular syndrome cases have been treated with shock wave for many years with variable results. I have seen some horses improve temporarily but have not seen any that have been "cured". Before treating the area, make sure you have an accurate diagnosis, use ultrasonographic guidance for placement of the probe. For DDFT insertional tears or enthesiopathy, use moderate to high setting at 1200-1500 shocks. Treatment area is either over the heel or through the frog depending on where the lesion is located.

ESWT machines produce strong acoustic waves when placed upon the tissue, including two mechanical forces: stress associated with the amplitude of the shock wave, and stresses and microjets associated with the expansion and collapse of cavitation bubbles. Complications associated with ESWT are caused by these stresses. The major problem is the acoustic cavitation and cavitation bubbles. When the tensile phase is large enough to pull the fluid apart, it creates cavitation bubbles. Cavititation is created when a micron size gas pocket is compressed by the acoustic wave and then enlarged by the tensile wave phase. The bubbles collapse, creating a high energy microjet of fluid that can damage tissue. Shock waves can also cause shear stress and tensile stresses in tissue which may help in breaking up calcification.Possible complications for the use of ESWT are few. If used in foals, they may develop swelling and petechiation (in white areas) when used at a high setting. We used ESWT in a foal with a cannon bone fracture, and he developed swelling over the area we shock waved. No skin was lost, but foals may need a lower setting then adult horses. Excessive energy or pulses may lead to tissue necrosis caused by cavitation of the cells. Shock waving areas with gas filled organs such as lungs, trachea, esophagus and intestines can lead to tissue damage and thus possible perforation. Air has low impedance, and the tissue surrounding it has fairly high impedance because of the amount of fluid in it. When the shock wave hits the tissue/air interface, almost all of the energy is reflected back to the tissue which can cause a high pressure build up causing tissue damage. The number one rule is never focus shock waves onto gas filled cavities or organs. Focusing shock waves onto large nerves and blood vessels may cause damage to vessel walls, thus causing arteries to rupture, leak or constrict. Just the expansion of the cavitation bubbles in the capillaries could cause tearing or rupture the vessels. Nerves may be damaged by cavitation and cause abnormal action potentials to form. High energy with extremely high numbers of shocks to bone may cause microfractures. Focusing shock waves onto cartilage may cause cartilage damage by lifting the cartilage from subchondral bone or damaging subchondral bone. Shock waving areas of neoplasia or infection may cause dispersement of neoplastic cells or bacteria. Shock waving the cervical vertebra is not recommended. The vertebral joints are closely associated with the spinal cord. The spinal cord can be seen with the ultrasound through the joints, and if you can ultrasound it you can hit it especially with shock waves. It is possible spinal cord damage could occur via cavitation of the cord, cavitational bubbles may occur in the subdural space, or vascular damage and inflammation in the subarchnoid area.

Conclusion

With all cases, a successful outcome to treatment starts with an accurate diagnosis. Imaging is vital to proper treatment. The days of "well it looks like the last one" diagnosis and then treatment with "bute and stall rest" should be long gone. Proper imaging is readily available via MRI, CT, digital ultrasound and radiographs. Stem cell therapy as well as ESWT is expensive, so treatments need to be more "pin pointed" if possible. Lameness treatment is expensive, inappropiate treatment is even more expensive. With stem cells and shockwave, many problems that had fair to guarded outcomes have good to excellent outcomes. Stem cell therapy is fast developing into the treatment of choice in many cases. It is an excellent supplement to go along with surgery but more research is still needed. ESWT has been around for several years but the manner in which it affects tissue still needs to be further investigated, but for now it is an excellent supplemental treatment.

References

[1] Alison M, Sarraf C. *Hepatic stem cells.* J Hepatol, 1998 Oct;29(4):676-82.

[2] Gage FH. *Mammalian neural stem cells.* Science, 2000 Feb 25;287(5457):1433-8.

[3] Weissman IL. *Translating stem and progenitor cell biology to the clinic: barriers and opportunities.* Science, 2000 Feb 25;287(5457):1442-6.

[4] De Bari C, Dell'Accio F, Tylzanowski P, Luyten FP. *Multipotent mesenchymal stem cells from adult human synovial membrane.* Arthritis Rheum, 2001 Aug;44(8):1928-42.

[5] Gronthos S, Franklin DM, Leddy HA, Robey PG, Storms RW, Gimble JM. *Surface protein characterization of human adipose tissue-derived stromal cells.* J Cell Physiol, 2001 Oct;189(1):54-63.

[6] Deasy BM, Jankowski RJ, Huard J. *Muscle-derived stem cells: characterization and potential for cell-mediated therapy.* Blood Cells Mol Dis, 2001 Sep-Oct;27(5):924-33.

[7] Hoynowski SM, Fry MM, Gardner BM, Leming MT, Tucker JR, Black L, et al. *Characterization and differentiation of equine umbilical cord-derived matrix cells.* Biochem Biophys Res Commun, 2007 Oct 19;362(2):347-53.

[8] Troyer DL, Weiss ML. *Wharton's jelly-derived cells are a primitive stromal cell population.* Stem Cells, 2008 Mar;26(3):591-9.

[9] Schaffler A, Buchler C. *Concise review: adipose tissue-derived stromal cells--basic and clinical implications for novel cell-based therapies.* Stem Cells, 2007 Apr;25(4):818-27.

[10] Thomson JA, Itskovitz-Eldor J, Shapiro SS, Waknitz MA, Swiergiel JJ, Marshall VS, et al. *Embryonic stem cell lines derived from human blastocysts.* Science, 1998 Nov 6;282(5391):1145-7.

[11] Guest DJ, Smith MR, Allen WR. *Monitoring the fate of autologous and allogeneic mesenchymal progenitor cells injected into the superficial digital flexor tendon of horses: preliminary study.* Equine Vet J, 2008 Mar;40(2):178-81.

[12] Rehman J, Traktuev D, Li J, Merfeld-Clauss S, Temm-Grove CJ, Bovenkerk JE, et al. *Secretion of angiogenic and antiapoptotic factors by human adipose stromal cells.* Circulation, 2004 Mar 16;109(10):1292-8.

[13] Nakagami H, Morishita R, Maeda K, Kikuchi Y, Ogihara T, Kaneda Y. *Adipose tissue-derived stromal cells as a novel option for regenerative cell therapy.* J Atheroscler Thromb, 2006 Apr;13(2):77-81.

[14] Nakagami H, Maeda K, Morishita R, Iguchi S, Nishikawa T, Takami Y, et al. *Novel autologous cell therapy in ischemic limb disease through growth factor secretion by cultured adipose tissue-derived stromal cells.* Arterioscler Thromb Vasc Biol, 2005 Dec;25(12):2542-7.

[15] Rehman J, Traktuev D, Li J, Merfeld-Clauss S, Temm-Grove CJ, Bovenkerk JE, et al. *Secretion of angiogenic and antiapoptotic factors by human adipose stromal cells.* Circulation, 2004 Mar 16;109(10):1292-8.

[16] Cao Y, Sun Z, Liao L, Meng Y, Han Q, Zhao RC. *Human adipose tissue-derived stem cells differentiate into endothelial cells in vitro and improve postnatal neovascularization in vivo.* Biochem Biophys Res Commun, 2005 Jul 1;332(2):370-9.

[17] Wang M, Crisostomo PR, Herring C, Meldrum KK, Meldrum DR. *Human progenitor cells from bone marrow or adipose tissue produce VEGF, HGF, and IGF-I in response to TNF by a p38 MAPK-dependent mechanism.* Am J Physiol Regul Integr Comp Physiol, 2006 Oct;291(4):R880-4.

[18] Kilroy GE, Foster SJ, Wu X, Ruiz J, Sherwood S, Heifetz A, et al. *Cytokine profile of human adipose-derived stem cells: expression of angiogenic, hematopoietic, and pro-inflammatory factors.* J Cell Physiol, 2007 Sep;212(3):702-9.

[19] Caplan AI, Dennis JE. *Mesenchymal stem cells as trophic mediators.* J Cell Biochem, 2006 Aug 1;98(5):1076-84.

[20] Murphy JM, Fink DJ, Hunziker EB, Barry FP. *Stem cell therapy in a caprine model of osteoarthritis.* Arthritis Rheum, 2003 Dec;48(12):3464-74.

[21] Schmidt M. *Neural stem cell differentiation factor discovered, Why neural stem cells divide and differentiate.* Goethe University Frankfurt. Release June 30, 2009; Available from: http://www.eurekalert.org/ pub_releases/2009-06/guf-nsc063009.php.

[22] Bakre MM, Hoi A, Mong JC, Koh YY, Wong KY, Stanton LW. *Generation of multipotential mesendodermal progenitors from mouse embryonic stem cells via sustained Wnt pathway activation.* J Biol Chem, 2007 Oct 26;282(43):31703-12.

[23] *Wnt signaling pathway.* [cited 2009]; Available from: http://en.wikipedia.org/wiki/Wnt_signaling_pathway.

[24] Casiraghi F, Azzollini N, Cassis P, Imberti B, Morigi M, Cugini D, et al. *Pretransplant infusion of mesenchymal stem cells prolongs the survival of a semiallogeneic heart transplant through the generation of regulatory T cells.* J Immunol, 2008 Sep 15;181(6):3933-46.

[25] Corcione A, Benvenuto F, Ferretti E, Giunti D, Cappiello V, Cazzanti F, et al. *Human mesenchymal stem cells modulate B-cell functions.* Blood, 2006 Jan 1;107(1):367-72.

[26] Rasmusson I. *Immune modulation by mesenchymal stem cells.* Exp Cell Res, 2006 Jul 15;312(12):2169-79.

[27] Meisel R, Zibert A, Laryea M, Gobel U, Daubener W, Dilloo D. *Human bone marrow stromal cells inhibit allogeneic T-cell responses by indoleamine 2,3-dioxygenase-mediated tryptophan degradation.* Blood, 2004 Jun 15;103(12):4619-21.

[28] Krampera M, Cosmi L, Angeli R, Pasini A, Liotta F, Andreini A, et al. *Role for interferon-gamma in the immunomodulatory activity of human bone marrow mesenchymal stem cells.* Stem Cells, 2006 Feb;24(2):386-98.

[29] Zhang W, Ge W, Li C, You S, Liao L, Han Q, et al. *Effects of mesenchymal stem cells on differentiation, maturation, and function of human monocyte-derived dendritic cells.* Stem Cells Dev, 2004 Jun;13(3):263-71.

[30] Aggarwal S, Pittenger MF. *Human mesenchymal stem cells modulate allogeneic immune cell responses.* Blood, 2005 Feb 15;105(4):1815-22.

[31] Koch TG, Berg LC, Betts DH. *Concepts for the clinical use of stem cells in equine medicine.* Can Vet J, 2008 Oct;49(10):1009-17.

[32] Genbacev O, Krtolica A, Zdravkovic T, Brunette E, Powell S, Nath A, et al. *Serum-free derivation of human embryonic stem cell lines on human placental fibroblast feeders.* Fertil Steril, 2005 May;83(5):1517-29.

[33] Xu C, Inokuma MS, Denham J, Golds K, Kundu P, Gold JD, et al. *Feeder-free growth of undifferentiated human embryonic stem cells.* Nat Biotechnol, 2001 Oct;19(10):971-4.

[34] Kern S, Eichler H, Stoeve J, Kluter H, Bieback K. *Comparative analysis of mesenchymal stem cells from bone marrow, umbilical cord blood, or adipose tissue.* Stem Cells, 2006 May;24(5):1294-301.

[35] Trippel SB, Ghivizzani SC, Nixon AJ. *Gene-based approaches for the repair of articular cartilage.* Gene Ther, 2004 Feb;11(4):351-9.

[36] Jorgensen C, Djouad F, Bouffi C, Mrugala D, Noel D. *Multipotent mesenchymal stromal cells in articular diseases.* Best Pract Res Clin Rheumatol, 2008 Apr;22(2):269-84.

[37] Stewart AA, Byron CR, Pondenis HC, Stewart MC. *Effect of dexamethasone supplementation on chondrogenesis of equine mesenchymal stem cells.* Am J Vet Res, 2008 Aug;69(8):1013-21.

[38] Sturtevant B. *Shock wave physics of lithotripters*. In: Smith AD, M.D. Smith's textbook of endourology. St. Louis, Mo.: Quality Medical Pub.; 1996.

[39] McClure SR, Van Sickle D, White MR. *Effects of extracorporeal shock wave therapy on bone*. Vet Surg, 2004 Jan-Feb;33(1):40-8.

[40] Ekkernkamp A, Haupt A, Knopf HJ, al. e. *Effects of extracorporeal shock waves on standardized fractures in sheep*. Urology, 1991;145:257-61.

[41] Suhr D, Brummer F, Hulser DF. *Cavitation-generated free radicals during shock wave exposure: investigations with cell-free solutions and suspended cells*. Ultrasound Med Biol, 1991;17(8):761-8.

[42] Johannes EJ, Kaulesar Sukul DM, Matura E. *High-energy shock waves for the treatment of nonunions: an experiment on dogs*. J Surg Res, 1994 Aug;57(2):246-52.

[43] Da Costa Gomez TM, Radtke CL, Kalscheur VL, Swain CA, Scollay MC, Edwards RB, et al. *Effect of focused and radial extracorporeal shock wave therapy on equine bone microdamage*. Vet Surg, 2004 Jan-Feb;33(1):49-55.

[44] Ohtori S, Inoue G, Mannoji C, Saisu T, Takahashi K, Mitsuhashi S, et al. *Shock wave application to rat skin induces degeneration and reinnervation of sensory nerve fibres*. Neurosci Lett, 2001 Nov 23;315(1-2):57-60.

[45] McClure S, Sonea IM, Yeager M, al. e. *Safety of shock wave therapy in performance horses*. Proc 49th Annu Conv Am Assoc Equine Pract, 2003;62:abstract.

[46] Bosch G, de Mos M, van Binsbergen R, van Schie HT, van de Lest CH, van Weeren PR. *The effect of focused extracorporeal shock wave therapy on collagen matrix and gene expression in normal tendons and ligaments*. Equine Vet J, 2009 Apr;41(4):335-41.

In: Rehabilitating the Athletic Horse
Editors: H. W. Jann et al., pp. 67-86
ISBN: 978-1-678-1-60876-672-7

Chapter 5

HYPERBARIC OXYGEN THERAPY

Dennis Geiser

DVM, Diplomate AVBP, Assistant Dean for Organizational Development and External Affairs, Associate Professor, Department of Large Animal Clinical SciencesCollege of Veterinary Medicine The University of Tennessee Knoxville, TN, USA

ABSTRACT

Five aspects of hyperbaric oxygen therapy are reviewed in this section; 1) the basic physical and physiologic principles that produce the desired increase in tissue oxygen concentrations, 2) the physiologic effects of hyperoxia, 3) indications for the use of hyperbaric oxygen as a primary or integrative therapy, 4) the potential application of hyperbaric oxygen in specific diseases including wounds, sepsis, bone healing and osteomyelitis, athletic injuries, reperfusion disease, blood loss, central nervous system diseases, carbon monoxide toxicity, 5) hyperbaric chambers and operation.

INTRODUCTION

Hyperbaric is defined as a higher than normal atmospheric pressure. Hyperbaric therapy occurs when a patient breaths a specific gas while experiencing a higher than normal atmospheric pressure on their body. Hyperbaric oxygen therapy (HBOT) would be defined as the breathing of oxygen while under a higher then normal atmospheric pressure. In most instances the patient would breathe 100% oxygen while under pressure. HBOT requires a means of creating a higher than normal pressure surrounding the patient. This is usually achieved through the use of a specialized chamber.

Hyperbaric therapy has its roots beginning in the 17th century. Two eras have been identified that led to modern day hyperbaric medicine, the compressed air era and the compressed oxygen era. Early experimentation with the use of either compressed air or oxygen occurred in the clinical setting, but lacked any reliable, controlled scientific basis or study. Many of the original theories on the effects of pressure were first developed and tested in the military setting and in response to the crippling "caisson disease" suffered by workers building underwater structures from a water tight chamber. Individuals like Paul Bert, Loraine Smith and JS Haldane developed early theories on the affect of pressure on the human body. It was not until 1955 that Ita Boerema, the Father of Modern HBOT, published evidence that pigs could live in a hyperbaric oxygen environment without red blood cells. In 1966 the US National Academy of Sciences' committee composed of members from the Navy and several universities produced a basic text called Fundamentals of Hyperbaric Medicine. In 1976 the Undersea Medical Society (UMS) became involved in clinical hyperbaric medicine and in 1977 another textbook appeared called Hyperbaric Oxygen Therapy. In 1986 the UMS changed its name to the Undersea and Hyperbaric Medical Society (UHMS). Since that time several hyperbaric medicine journals have been published, physician and nurse certification programs have been created, and training programs have been established. Research in hyperbaric therapy now contributes to the development of indications for HBOT and the associated clinical therapy protocols.

THE PHYSICS OF PRESSURE

Terminology

Pressure is defined as force per unit area. In the case of gases, the pressure that a gas exerts is caused by the number of gas molecules moving around and exerting a force on a body surface or other container. At sea level a body experiences a pressure caused by the weight of a column of air extending into the atmosphere. The pressure at sea level exerted by the atmosphere is 14.7 $lb/in.^2$ (psi), 760 mmHg, 0.99 BAR, or 1 atmosphere absolute (ATA). Descending below sea level and ascending into the atmosphere increases and decreases the size of the air column and therefore increases or decreases the pressure exerted respectively. Water is denser and weighs more than air because it contains more molecules per unit volume than air and therefore exerts a greater pressure than air for the same column height. Thirty three feet of salt water (fsw) exerts the same pressure on the body as the column of atmospheric air at sea level, 14.7 psi, 760 mmHg, or 1 ATA. For every additional 33 fsw increase in depth another 14.7 psi or 1 ATA of pressure is added (Figure 1).

Pressure (psi)	Feet of sea water	Atmospheres Absolute	Relative Volume	Relative Density
14.7	sea level	1 ATA	1	1
29.4	33	2 ATA	1/2	2
44.1	66	3 ATA	1/3	3
58.8	99	4 ATA	1/4	4
73.5	132	5 ATA	1/5	5

Figure 1. Absolute pressure and the effect of pressure on air space volume and gas density.

Absolute pressure is the total pressure that a patient is experiencing and always includes atmospheric pressure plus the gauge pressure. The same effect is created in the hyperbaric chamber by the addition of gas (air or oxygen) into a closed container (chamber) in which the patient is placed. Each treatment is similar to performing a scuba dive to a certain depth and is often called "a dive".

Gas Laws

Four gas laws can be used to explain the ability of hyperbaric oxygen or air therapy to significantly increase the arterial and tissue oxygen content; Boyles, Henry's, Dalton's, and Grahm's Laws (Figure 2).

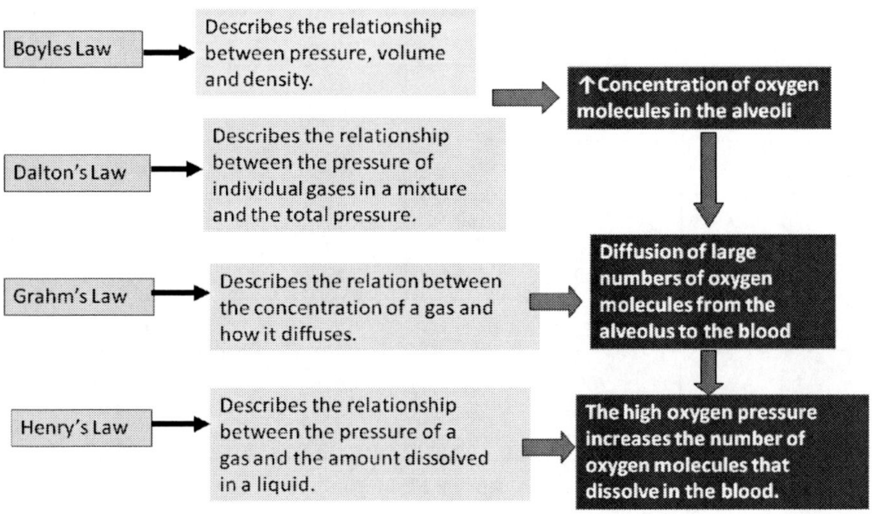

Figure 2. Physical gas laws that explain the blood and tissue hyperoxia produced by HBOT.

Boyles Law

As the pressure around a patient increases the volume of any gas filled space in the body decreases including each pulmonary alveolus. As the volume decreases the gas molecules in the space are concentrated or become denser. So as the volume decreases the density increases. Because of Boyle's Law the application of hyperbaric therapy increases the oxygen molecule density in each alveolus, presenting more oxygen molecules for diffusion across the alveolar - capillary interface and into the blood (Figures 1 and 2).

Dalton's Law

In a mixture of gases the pressure of each individual gas contributes to the total pressure exerted by the gas (the whole is a sum of its parts). The air we breath is essentially 21% O_2,

78% N_2, and 1 % other gases. For this chapterwe will use 21% O_2 and 79% N_2. Together the sum of this mixture of two gases equal 100%. The percentage of each gas multiplied times the total pressure would equal the partial pressure of the individual gas in the mixture. At sea level the pressure of oxygen in mmHg would be 760 mmHg x 0.21 = 159.6 mmHg and the pressure of nitrogen would be 760 mmHg x .79 = 600.4 mmHg. The total, 159.6 + 600.4 = 760 mmHg. If the percentage of one of the gases in the mixture is increased or if the total pressure surrounding the patient is increased then the pressure of the individual gas or gases in the mixture will increase. Breathing 100% O_2 at sea level yields 760 mmHg x 1.0 = 760 mmHg oxygen, over 4.5 times the oxygen pressure when breathing air at sea level. If the total surrounding pressure increases then the pressure of the individual gas also increase. If a patient breaths 100% O_2 at 2 ATA this would yield 1520 mmHg x 1.0 = 1520 mmHg oxygen (Figure 3).

Inhaled Gas			In the Lung	In the Plasma
Total Pressure [ATA]	Total Pressure [mmHg]	PO_2 [mmHg]	P_AO_2 [mmHg]	ml O_2/dl blood [vol%]
Breathing Air				
1	760	160	100	0.31
2	1520	319	269	0.83
3	2280	479	429	1.33
Breathing 100% O_2				14.32 x
1	760	760	673	2.06
2	1520	1520	1433	4.44
3	2280	2280	2056	5.80

Breathing 100% oxygen at 2 ATA delivers 15 times more oxygen to the tissues as breathing room air

Figure 3. The approximate values for oxygen concentrations in inspired gases, alveolar gases and plasma under normobaric and hyperbaric conditions breathing air and 100% oxygen.

Graham's Law

Grahm's Law and Fick's Law describe the relationship of the pressure (concentration) of a gas and how it moves from one area to another. In the lung gases must diffuse across a semi-permeable membrane that includes the alveolar wall a very small interstitial space and the capillary wall. Oxygen in the alveolus is continuously replenished by respiratory efforts moving the inhaled gases to the alveoli. Blood returning from the tissues has had oxygen extracted and the concentration decreases below that of the arterial blood. This sets up a pressure gradient such that the venous oxygen pressure is lower than that of the alveolus and oxygen then diffuses to area of lower concentration as described by Grahm's Law (Figure 3).

If we increase the concentration of oxygen molecules in the alveolus, as occurs with hyperbaric therapy (via Boyles and Dalton's Laws), even more oxygen will be available to move across the alveolar-capillary interface. The same law of diffusion applies at the tissue level. However, in some cases the diffusion distance is considerably greater. Tissue oxygen is affected by the fractional inspired oxygen concentration (FiO_2), cardiac output, blood flow, cellular metabolism (O_2 consumption), and substrate availability. Tissue oxygen content depends on the concentration gradient and the diffusion distance. Oxygen diffusion decreases by a three fold factor as the distance increases. A twenty fold increase in capillary oxygen content increases the diffusion distance four fold. Hyperbaric oxygen therapy elevates the blood oxygen content which causes oxygen to diffuse farther from the capillaries.

Henry's Law

Henry's law relates the pressure of a gas to how much of that gas can be dissolved (solubility) in a liquid. In the case of the body the liquid is the blood. The gas pressure is the pressure of oxygen as it diffuses from the alveolus to the blood. Following the diffusion of oxygen into the blood, a certain amount is immediately combined with hemoglobin (ceiling affect). Ninety seven percent of a patient's hemoglobin will be saturated when breathing air at sea level with a very small amount of oxygen dissolved in the plasma (oxyhemoglobin dissociation curve). The **oxygen capacity** of the blood is the maximum amount of oxygen that can be combined with hemoglobin. One gram of hemoglobin combines with 1.36 ml of oxygen. If the blood contains 15 g/dl of hemoglobin then 1 dl of blood transports approximately 20.4 ml of oxygen as oxyhemoglobin. Approximately 0.0031 ml of oxygen can be dissolved in each decaliter of plasma for every mmHg pressure of oxygen. At 100 mmHg O_2 pressure, 1 ATA, 0.31 ml/dl oxygen will be dissolved in the plasma. The **oxygen content** is the total amount of oxygen in the blood; oxygen combined with hemoglobin plus dissolved oxygen.

Breathing 100% oxygen at 1 ATA will completely saturate hemoglobin and increase the amount of oxygen dissolved in the plasma. For each increase in absolute pressure more oxygen will dissolve in the plasma (Figure 3).

PHYSIOLOGY OF PRESSURE

Knowledge of hyperbaric therapy must include information on the potential effects of pressure on the body. In the diving industry these affects are often categorized into direct and indirect affects.

The Direct Effects of Pressure

The direct affects of pressure are termed barotraumas and include squeezes, blocks and pulmonary trauma. Squeezes and blocks are related to the effects of pressure on gas filled spaces as described by Boyle's Law and the contraction and expansion of air filled spaces on descent and ascent. The most common squeeze in humans is an ear squeeze when the pressure on either side of the tympanic membrane fails to equalize as the surrounding pressure increases. The effect is the same as that felt when ascending and descending in an aircraft.

Failure to equalize the pressure on the tympanic membrane can result in severe pain and eventually rupture of the membrane. Other common sites for squeezes and blocks include the sinuses, intestines and dental fillings. It is not clear whether animals experience the pressure effects in their ears and the effect of hyperbaric therapy on the eustachian tube and the equine guttural pouches. A sinus block occurs when air within the sinus is unable to escape upon ascent due to swelling or some other obstruction. The production of excessive gas in the intestinal tract that was not present during descent may produce abdominal pain upon ascent as the pressure decreases and the gas expands.

Pulmonary barotrauma occurs when gas in the lungs cannot adequately escape to maintain a normal volume and pressure as the patient ascends from high to lower pressure. In divers this occurs for two major reasons, breath holding on ascent or ascending too rapidly. It is imperative that patients exhale at a normal rate during ascent from a pressurized treatment or when scuba diving. There are four major syndromes associated with pulmonary barotraumas; 1) subcutaneous emphysema, 2) pneumomediastinum, 3) pneumothorax, and 4) arterial gas embolism (AGE). It is not anticipated that animal patients would breath hold during therapy. However, with some lung diseases that produce a pneumothorax, hyperbaric therapy may produce a tension pneumothorax on ascent from depth if an exit path for thoracic or mediastinal air is not present.

The Indirect Effects of Pressure

The indirect effects of pressure include decompression sickness (DCS), nitrogen narcosis, and oxygen toxicity. Traditionally, divers utilize compressed air as their breathing mixture. Because air is nitrogen rich (and 79%) and nitrogen is an inert gas, breathing air under pressure delivers a large amount of nitrogen to the blood and tissue. As the pressure is reduced (ascent) nitrogen comes out of the tissues and returns to the blood to be removed via the lungs. Bubbles of nitrogen have been detected in divers even when DCS has not occurred. If the ascent is too rapid without adequate off-gassing or if large amounts of nitrogen have accumulated in the tissue because of the completion of multiple dives without adequate surface time to permit expulsion of the tissue nitrogen the risk of DCS increases. Bubbles may then enlarge according to Boyle's Law as the surrounding pressure decreases. These bubbles then accumulate in small capillaries throughout the body. Decompression sickness is manifested by several clinical syndromes. In animal hyperbaric therapy most chambers utilize 100% oxygen as the breathing and pressurizing gas. There are some chambers, similar to multi-place chambers in human hyperbaric therapy, that utilize air for pressurization while the patient breaths 100% oxygen by mask. If the breathing gas is 100% oxygen the possibility of inducing DCS is minimal if not eliminated.

Nitrogen narcosis is a syndrome that is also due to the accumulation of nitrogen in the body as depth and pressure increases. In humans it is initially evident at approximately 90-100 fsw ($\approx$ 3 ATA). Nitrogen narcosis reduces mental and motor ability and impairs judgment and orientation. As with DCS, narcosis due to nitrogen should not be a concern for patients in the 100% oxygen environment of the hyperbaric chamber.

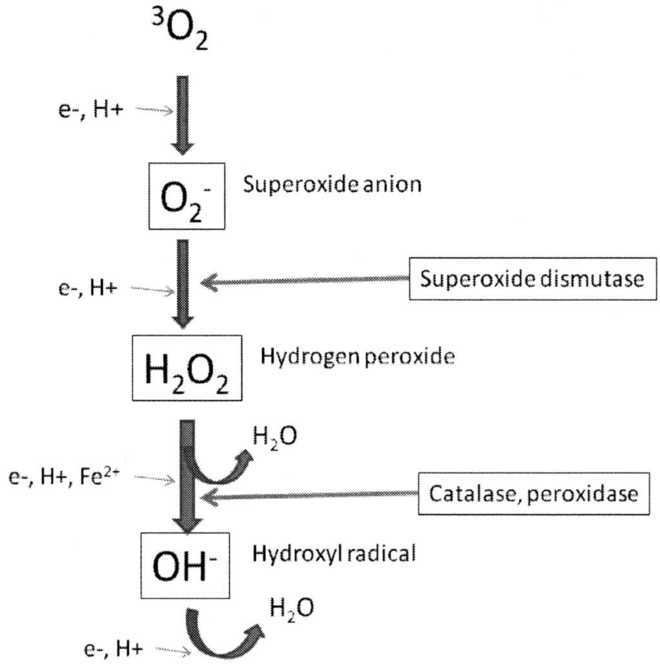

Figure 4. Cascade for the generation of oxygen radicals.

Oxygen toxicity is a concern in HBOT. Although oxygen is an active compound in the body that is continually utilized in tissue function, oxygen can reach levels that are toxic to a patient. Consequently, in HBOT, oxygen is considered a drug and as such has specific doses and frequency and duration of application. The formation of reactive oxygen species (ROS) during hyperoxic therapy is considered the cause of oxygen toxicity and associated tissue reactions (Figure 4). However, the potent antioxidant defense mechanisms of the body make hyperbaric oxygen therapy a safe, therapeutic modality. Only when those defense mechanisms are overwhelmed because of exposure to oxygen at high pressures (> 3 ATA) or because of prolonged exposure will the risk of oxygen toxicity increase. Reactive oxygen species produce lipid peroxidation, protein oxidation, and enzyme inactivation. The body's defense mechanism against ROS production includes superoxide dismutase (SOD), catalase, glutathione reductase and peroxidase, and enzymes associated with the pentose phosphate pathway. Vitamin C and E, selenium and glutathione also have potent antioxidant capacities. The degree of ROS damage is a function of the balance or imbalance between antioxidants and ROS production.

Oxygen toxicity is usually manifested in either the central nervous system (CNS) or the pulmonary system. CNS toxicity is manifested by grand mal seizures which can be pre-empted by signs that include sweating, bradycardia, depression, apprehension, inspiratory predominance, nausea and vomiting, and twitching of the lips, cheek, nose or eyelids. When the patient is switched to air, signs usually subside without lasting untoward effects, except for physical trauma that may occur during a seizure.

Pulmonary oxygen toxicity produces a syndrome similar to adult respiratory distress syndrome. Tracheal and bronchial irritation eventually lead to coughing and dyspnea with progressive impairment of pulmonary function. The initial pathology associated with pulmonary toxicity is reversible. Continued exposure to oxygen without appropriate intervals of air breathing can result in the cumulative effects. The degree of pulmonary intoxication has been quantified using the concept of a unit pulmonary toxic dose (UPTD). Oxygen toxicity does occur in animals who are administered long term, 100% oxygen therapy. Hyperbaric treatment protocols that might produce oxygen toxicity in the various animal species are yet to be determined as is any quantification of pulmonary toxicity. In multi-place human chambers, pressurized with air, patients can easily receive alternate 100% oxygen and air treatments to reduce the potential of oxygen toxicity.

TISSUE OXYGENATION

Improved tissue oxygenation is the ultimate goal of hyperbaric therapy. Tissue oxygen concentrations are influenced by the inspired concentration of oxygen (F_iO_2), cardiac output, tissue blood flow, and cellular metabolism (consumption). Diffusion of oxygen from the blood to the cells depends on the concentration gradient and the distance the cell is from the capillary, diffusion distance. The distance an oxygen molecule will diffuse is proportional to the square root of the capillary oxygen content. A 20 fold increase in PO_2 increases the diffusion distance approximately four fold. Adenosine triphosphate formation requires a minimum of 0.5-3.0 mmHg of oxygen in the mitochondria which correlates to a minimum of 30 mmHg oxygen in the tissue. Many compromised tissues (chronic wounds, osteomyelitis, flaps, etc.) will have an oxygen concentration less than 30 mmHg. The ability of hyperbaric oxygen therapy to increase blood oxygen concentrations by 15-20 times normal values significantly improves the oxygen diffusion distance in the tissues.

The Physiologic and Therapeutic Effects of Hyperbaric Oxygen

Oxygen should be considered as a drug and as such has specific dosages, durations and frequencies of administration, a therapeutic index, minimum effective concentration, and a minimum toxic concentration. A specific dose response should be considered for oxygen as with any other therapeutic agent. Some of the general physiologic affects of hyperbaric oxygen therapy are summarized in Figure 5.

Hyperbaric oxygen therapy is part of an “integrative medicine” program and can be both a primary and an adjunctive therapy in the treatment of disease. Initially, HBOT was utilized as a primary therapy for decompression sickness and arterial gas embolism. Hyperbaric therapy is considered a primary treatment for carbon monoxide and cyanide toxicity, and anaerobic bacterial disease, specifically Clostridium perfringens infections. In human medicine the availability of third party payment for medical and surgical procedures significantly affects the list of acceptable applications of HBOT. The use of HBOT for diseases outside of those acceptable is usually investigational or patient financed. In veterinary medicine we are able to apply HBOT in many diseases.

Some of the indications for the use of HBOT as a primary or complimentary and adjunctive therapy are listed in Figure 6.

- Reduction in tissue and vascular gas bubble size.
- Reduction in inert gas accumulation due to breathing various gas mixture at pressure
- Increase plasma dissolved oxygen to levels sufficient to meet body needs and life.
- Increased diffusion of oxygen into the tissues.
- Slight decrease in blood pH: Hb is oxygen saturated causing an increase in dissolved CO_2.
- Reduction in blood flow in hyperoxic and normoxic tissues, increased or no change in blood flow in hypoxic tissues.
- Gradual decrease in CBF as O_2 increased up to 2 ATA, greater than 2 ATA CBF decreases.
- Increase in anti-oxidant production
- Decreased lipid peroxidation.
- Modulates nitric oxide production.
- Decreases edema
- Hyperoxia decreased blood flow in myocardium, kidney, ocular globe, and splanchnic areas in rats, decrease cardiac output with increase in afterload in man.
- Stimulation of collagen production.
- Stimulation of osteoclastic activity.
- Decreased Hct, platelet aggregation, & WBC adherence.
- Modifies growth factors.
- Simulate capillary budding.
- Promotes cell proliferation
- Tissue salvage (peripheral ischemias & reperfusion, burns, radiation therapy, viability of tissue flaps)
- Transient myopia

Figure 5. Some general physiologic effects of HBOT.

Hyperbaric Oxygen Therapy and Infection

Increasing oxygen tensions in tissues invaded by an infectious agent may have a variety of affects on the infectious agent. Hyperoxia and hyperbaric oxygen may be bacteriocidal or static depending on the tissue oxygen concentration and ability of the organism to produce antioxidants. In most cases the direct affects of hyperbaric therapy in bacterial inhibition are mediated through the production of reactive oxygen species (ROS). In some cases hyperoxia will promote the growth of aerobic bacteria. The indirect affects of hyperbaric oxygen and hyperoxia on infectious agents include; 1) support of neutrophilic killing of organism by oxidative burst, 2) augmentation of antimicrobial affects, 3) improving infected tissue repair and return to function. In the horse HBOT has been successfully utilized in a wide variety of infectious processes including Rhodococcus equi pneumonia, septic arthritis, pleuritis, osteomyelitis, Clostridial diseases, septic tendonitis, abdominal abscesses, and others.

Anaerobic bacteria are susceptible to hyperbaric oxygen because they are unable to provide antioxidant defenses against ROS. Oxygen is bacteriocidal for *Clostridium perfringens* in vitro at a high pressure for extended exposure times. At acceptable therapy levels hyperoxic conditions may prevent Clostridial spore germination. Facultative anaerobic bacteria may grow in hyperoxic conditions if they can develop the production of antioxidants. In some cases, hyperoxia, but not HBOT, will enhance aerobic bacterial growth. The cidal or static affect of hyperbaric conditions on aerobic bacteria depend on pressure and time of treatment. Many studies have been completed under *in vitro* conditions and required pressures and treatment times are in excess of those clinically acceptable. Hyperbaric therapy affects the growth of bacteria through several mechanism; 1) inhibition of amino acid and protein synthesis, 2) decreasing concentration of metabolic co-factors, 3) blocking DNA synthesis or increasing its degradation, 4) increase of ROS production.

White blood cells are capable of phagocytosis in both normoxic and hypoxic environments. Neutrophils are capable of killing bacteria intracellularly and extracellularly, through oxygen dependent and oxygen independent mechanisms. The oxygen dependent mechanism requires that significant amounts of oxygen be available to produce several ROSs involved in bacterial killing. The ROS include superoxide anion, hydrogen peroxide, hydrochlorous acid, hydroxide anion, and hydroxyl radical. Hyperbaric therapy and resulting hyperoxia is particularly beneficial in improving oxidative bacterial killing in hypoxic and otherwise compromised tissues.

The affects of oxygen tensions and hyperbaric conditions on antimicrobials depend on the type of bacterial agent and the mechanism of action of the antibiotic.

Hypoxia and anoxia (anaerobic conditions) will decrease the activity of some antibiotics. Most studies that investigate the role of oxygen in antimicrobial effectiveness have been performed in vitro by determining MIC against various organisms. For example, the MIC of aminoglycoside antibiotics, in anaerobic conditions, is increased against *E. coli, Klebsiella, Salmonella, Staphylococcus,* and *Streptococcus* species. Low oxygen tensions appear to decrease the transport of aminoglycosides into the bacteria. Other antimicrobials whose activity is affected by oxygen tensions include sulfamethoxazole, trimethoprim, vancomycin, fluoroquinilones, cephalosporins, streptomycin, and rifampin. In most cases the activity of the antimicrobial is not completely inhibited by low oxygen tensions but normoxic and hyperoxic conditions improve the activity.

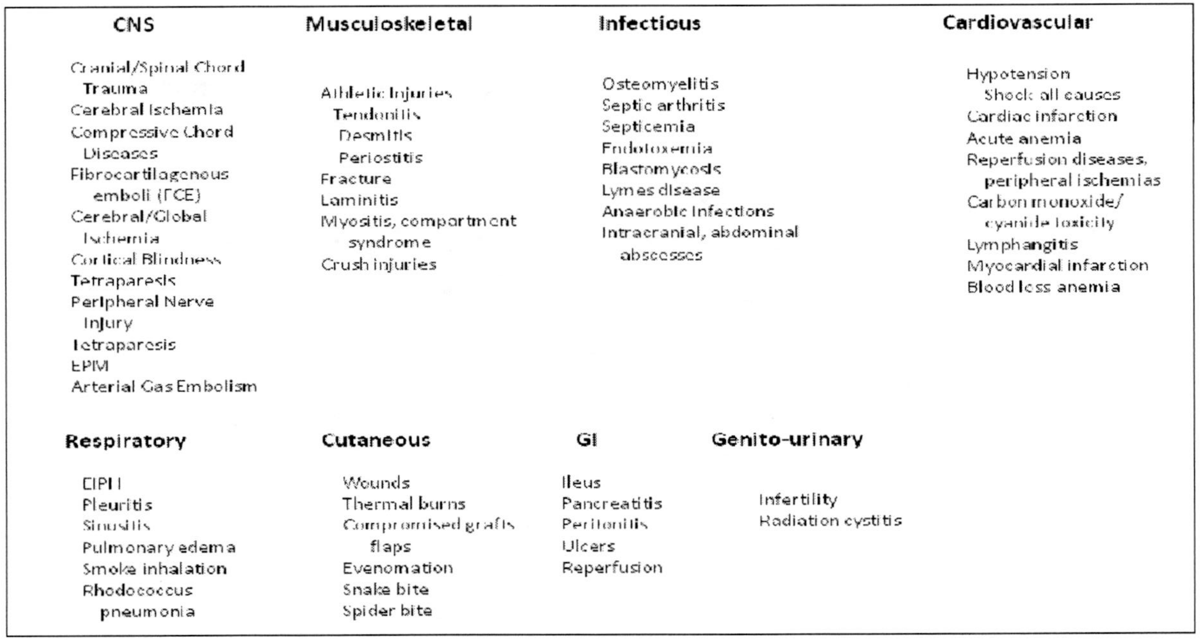

Figure 6. Some, but not all, of the potential indications for the use of HBOT in veterinary medicine.

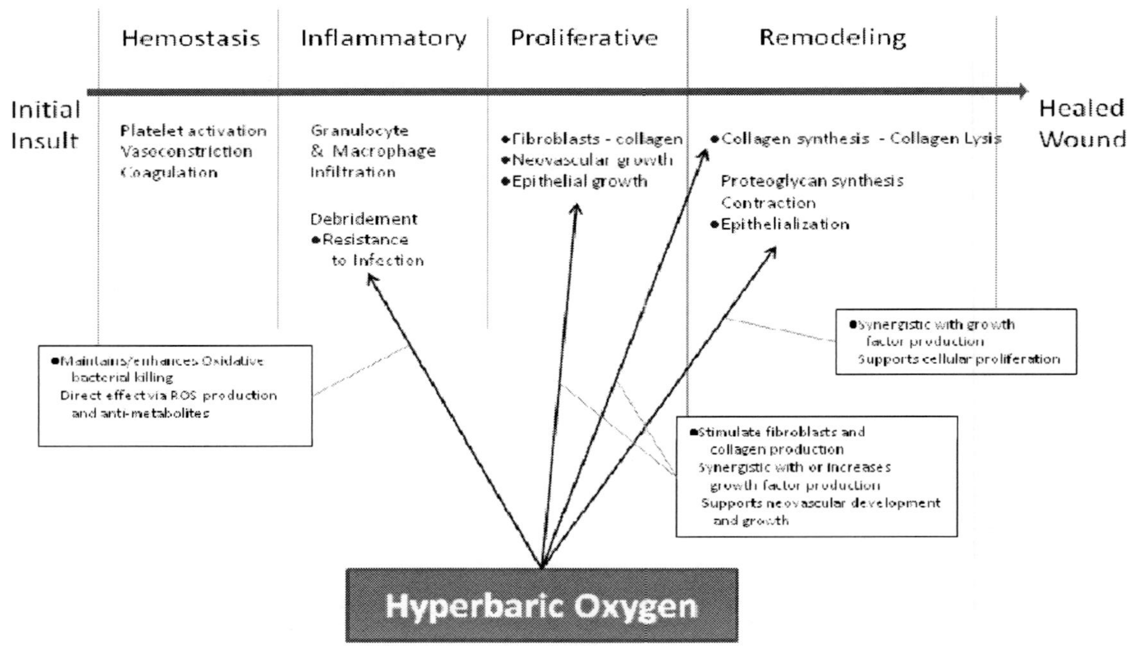

Figure 7. The effect of HBOT on the various stages of wound healing.

Increased oxygen tensions may potentiate the activity of antibiotics by several mechanism; 1) reversing anaerobic or hypoxic conditions, 2) increasing the post antibiotic effect (PAE), 3) potentiating the antimetabolite activity of antibiotics, 4) enhancing oxidation-reduction cycling, 5) enhancing antimicrobial metabolic activation. Most studies have focused on *in vitro* models and results may be different *in vivo*. The effects of hyperbaric therapy on bacterial organisms encountered in the horse are yet to be determined.

Hyperbaric Oxygen Therapy and Wound Healing

The most frequent application of hyperbaric oxygen in human medicine, in addition to the treatment of diving related problems, occurs in the management of compromised wounds and particularly for the healing of wounds of diabetic patients.

Although hyperbaric oxygen therapy will aid in the healing of any wound, it has its most efficacious application in the healing of wounds impaired by hypo-perfusion and ischemia, tissue hypoxia, and infection. Adjunct hyperbaric oxygen therapy improves healing in a variety of wounds that occur from crush injuries, severe tissue necrosis, infections (osteomyelitis, soft tissue infections), wounds with vascular compromise, wounds with compromised or failing skin flaps or grafts, burns, and tissue injury resulting from radiation.

The major deterrents to wound healing are hypo-perfusion, tissue hypoxia and infection. The equine distal limb presents an excellent physiologic environment for the creation of a compromised wound due to the lack of significant soft tissue structures and their associated vascular supply. Hypo-perfusion and hypoxia contribute to decreased wound healing by decreasing fibroblastic proliferation, decreased collagen production, impaired capillary angiogenesis, and the decreased ability to control infection. Hyperbaric oxygen therapy restores oxygen tensions in hypo-perfused wounds by significantly increasing the oxygen tension in the blood that does reach the wound and by creating an improved blood to tissue oxygen gradient that increases the distance oxygen will diffuse into the wounded tissues. The effects of HBOT on compromised wounds are summarized in Figure 7.

Healthy wounds heal through a series of events orchestrated by the cellular response, leading to the production of chemotactants, inflammatory mediators, and growth factors. In the healthy wound environmental lactate concentrations, an initial tissue hypoxia, and nitrous oxide concentrations stimulate the events leading to angiogenesis, arborization of capillaries and granulation tissue formation. Opponents to the use of HBOT point out that increasing the oxygen level in the wound by hyperbaric therapy eliminates the stimulus of elevated lactate and hypoxia and therefore is not beneficial and may be detrimental. However, in compromised wounds, chronic wounds, and large wounds the initial hypoxic stimulus for the repair process continues to be present do to severe vascular compromise and HBOT will play a significant role in promoting and accelerating the healing process. Continued and constant hypoxia contributes to the decreased production, inhibition, and increased degradation of growth factors (Figure 8) that are crucial in the repair process. In healthy wounds and grafts the **intermittent** (every other day) application of HBOT will help reverse the hypoxia and accelerate healing while maintaining periods of low oxygen tensions to stimulate angiogenesis. HBOT increases the production or decreases the degradation of some growth factors and acts synergistically with others to increase the rate of healing. The intermittent use allows for periods of hypoxia that might occur naturally in healthy wounds not exposed to hyperbaric oxygen. Hyperbaric oxygen therapy is effective in the control of infection in wounded tissues through the support of oxidative killing and other mechanisms discussed in the previous section.

Growth Factors	HBOT Effect	Result
Vascular Endothelial Growth Factor [VEGF]	↑ production	↑ angiogenesis ↑ capillary arborization ↑ granulation formation
Platelet derived Growth Factor [PDGF]	Facilitates the effects	↑ stimulation of fibroblast to secrete collagen ↑ attraction of mesenchymal cells
Fibroblastic Growth Factor [FGF]	Synergistic with FGF in ischemic wounds	↑ angiogenesis ↑ attraction of mesenchymal cells

Figure 8. A summary of some of the effects of hyperoxia on tissue growth factors.

Hyperbaric Oxygen Therapy and Ischemia and Reperfusion Disease

Reperfusion disease is characterized by accelerated microcirculatory injury resulting in cell death caused by reperfusion and the infusion of oxygen following prolonged periods of ischemia. Some of the clinical syndromes that occur in equine medicine that may involve reperfusion disease are the surgical repair of intestinal obstruction (volvulus, torsion), treatment of exertional myopathy (compartment syndrome), and laminitis. Other situations that may initiate reperfusion disease include failing skin flaps, high impact trauma and crush injuries, cerebral ischemia, and cardiac disease. Excessive oxygen radical production and progressive, persistent vasoconstriction is theorized as the major cause of cell damage in reperfusion disease. Superoxide anion (O_2^-) and hydroxyl radical (OH^-) are two of the common radicals involved and are generated through the hypoxanthine-xanthine – xanthine oxidase system in capillary endothelial cells during reperfusion. These unstable radicals lead to lipid peroxidation causing cell death. The second source of oxygen radicals is the activated neutrophil. Following severe, prolonged ischemia, reperfusion produces an initial vasodilation followed by a severe vasoconstriction of the microcirculation. The increased adherence of neutrophils to the endothelial cells of post capillary venules following reperfusion and the release of oxygen radicals initiates disruption of the basement membrane of the venule. It is theorized that vasoactive substances released into the interstitium will then affect local arterioles resulting in vasoconstriction and further prolonged ischemia. Numerous studies have confirmed the increased neutrophil adhesion and venule disruption as well as the flow characteristics of the microcirculation following reperfusion. Several substances promote neutrophil adherence including TNF, interleukins, complement, chemotactic substances, platelet activating factor and oxygen radicals.

Investigators and clinicians were initially concerned that HBOT would exacerbate the microvascular affects of reperfusion disease by the creation of additional free radicals. Several studies have shown improvement in microvascular blood flow and increased survivability of skin flaps treated with HBOT following reperfusion disease. Studies have shown that the use of HBOT in reperfusion disease in experimentally created compartment syndrome in dogs and mice decreased skeletal muscle edema and necrosis. In a rat gracilis muscle model of reperfusion, HBOT decreased leukocyte adherence and prevented arteriolar vasoconstriction when compared to untreated subjects. Initial studies indicate that the timing of HBOT therapy is important and should occur within 1-4 hrs. after reperfusion. When an ischemic episode exceeds 6 hrs. permanent damage may occur despite HBOT. As with many therapies, the earlier the application of the appropriate therapy the better the results. In the laminitis syndrome this is particularly true. There is some evidence that reperfusion disease may play a roll in the development of laminitis. HBOT applied in the developmental (prodromal) and in the acute phases may be beneficial. Identifying patients at a high risk of developing laminitis and treating with HBOT "may" prevent the onset of the disease. Other syndromes that occur in the horse include myositis/compartment syndrome, intestinal ischemia, and ischemia of grafts and flaps, cerebral trauma and ischemia. Hyperbaric oxygen therapy after abdominal, intestinal surgery may help salvage and revitalize compromised tissue. There are some indications that HBOT may also be beneficial in preventing or treating ileus.

Hyperbaric oxygen therapy prevents or diminishes the severity of ischemia-reperfusion by blocking neutrophil adhesion in post-arteriolar venules and by increasing the production of oxygen radical scavengers. The effects of ischemia-reperfusion and the effect of HBOT are summarized in Figure 9. As with many therapies the earlier the application of the appropriate therapy the better the results

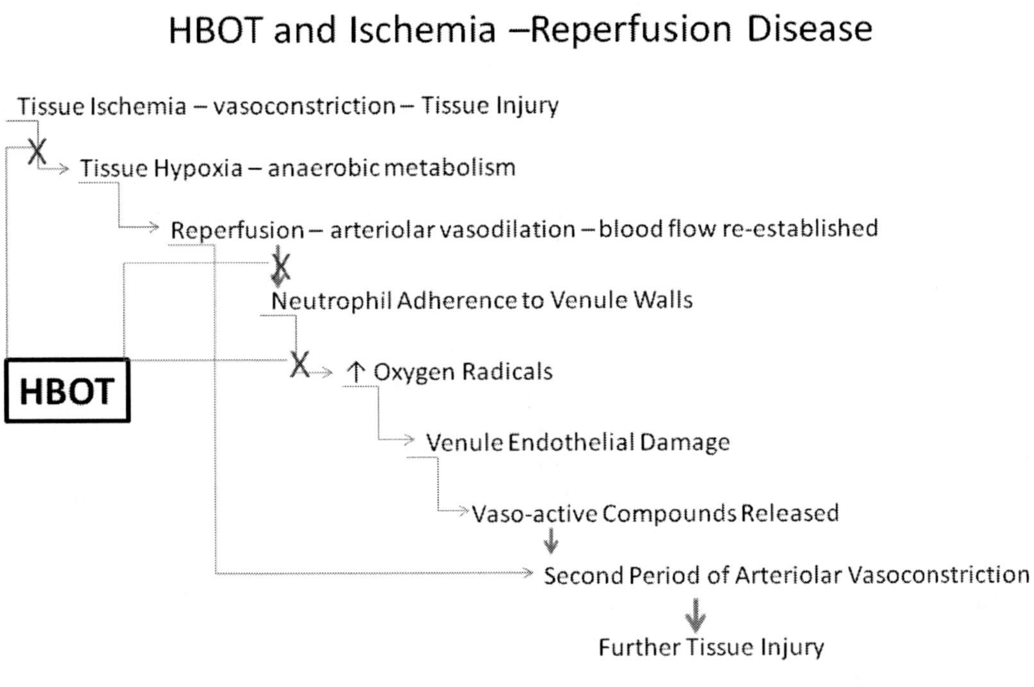

Figure 9. The effects of HBOT in preventing and treating reperfusion disease.

Hyperbaric Oxygen Therapy and Neurologic Disease and Head Trauma

Anaerobic metabolism in neural tissue leads to acidosis and energy depletion, loss of cellular homeostasis and ionic balance. Intracellular proteases are activated and oxygen radical production ensues that will result in additional cell damage and loss. Hyperbaric therapy is beneficial in cerebral ischemia, cerebral edema, and peripheral neuropathies due to trauma and ischemia. The benefit attained from HBOT is the provision of oxygen to reverse acidosis and resuscitate cells that are compromised but not permanently damaged. In cerebral disease, the increased oxygen produces cerebral vasoconstriction and reduces CBF as long as cerebral autoregulation is intact. Vasoconstriction contributes to the reduction of edema in diseased and traumatized neural tissues. In veterinary medicine hyperbaric therapy has been used in a wide range of neurologic diseases in small animals with only a few anecdotal reports (EPM, head trauma, cortical blindness) on its use in large animals (Figure 6). Reports are available in the literature on use of HBOT in controlled neurologic research and clinical neurologic disease.

Hyperbaric Oxygen Therapy and Bone Repair and Osteomyelitis

Bone repair is based on both resorption (osteoclasts) and deposition (osteoblasts) of the boney matrix. Hyperbaric oxygen therapy stimulates osteoclastic activity that leads to bone resorption and remodeling. This phenomenon may be due to an increase in oxygen radical production adjacent to bone surfaces. Several studies using laboratory animal models have indicated accelerated vascular in growth, increased collagen matrix and bone deposition, increased bone mineral density and torsional strength following appropriate hyperbaric therapy. The trauma that occurs from fractures of the distal equine limb produces significant vascular compromise in an area where there is already a lack of soft tissue and vascular support. Even in a non-infected fracture, bone oxygen tensions can be reduced to the point that the normal repair cycle is compromised which slows healing and impairs protective mechanisms against bacterial infection. HBOT has been utilized in the successful treatment of acute and chronic septic arthritis and physitis in conjunction with antimicrobial and antiinflammatory therapy.

Hyperbaric therapy has been shown to be beneficial for the treatment of refractory osteomyelitis in both human clinical trials and laboratory animal models.

Studies have shown that HBOT increases oxygen tension in both infected and non-infected bone. Oxygen tensions in bone of < 25 mmHg are not conducive to healing or to maintenance of antibacterial defenses. The mechanisms through which HBOT is beneficial in osteomyelitis are the same as those described under infection above; 1) increased phagocytic killing, 2) bacteriocidal affects on anaerobic and microaerophilic organisms, 3) enhancement of antimicrobial effectiveness, 4) edema and inflammation reduction. HBOT also restores fibroblastic activity and collagen matrix production in hypoxic tissue and supports the restoration of the resorption/deposition cycle.

The duration, frequency and dose of hyperbaric oxygen determine if a positive or negative affect is produced in patients with osteomyelitis. In rat models treatment at 2-3 ATA, for 90-120 minutes, once daily was optimal. Excessive treatment and inadequate treatment resulted in excessive bone resorption and more collagen deposition, and inhibition of the remodeling cycle and defense mechanisms respectively.

HBOT has been utilized in the successful treatment of horses with acute and chronic septic arthritis and physitis in conjunction with antimicrobial and antiinflammatory therapy.

Hyperbaric Oxygen Therapy and Athletic Injuries

There are a variety of performance induced injuries that occur in the horse. From the standpoint of integrative medicine, HBOT, in conjunction with conventional therapies, can provide more functional healing in a shorter period of time. Anecdotal case reports have shown a benefit of HBOT in MC III periostitis, acute and chronic suspensory desmitis and flexor tendonitis, bone cysts, cartilage defects, sesamoiditis, myositis, and post fracture repair. The author has been involved in the management of three to four horses with severe suspensory desmitis (including one case of bilateral core rear suspensory lesions). The combination of local, fat derived stem cells followed by HBOT produced excellent results with better tendon fiber alignment and shorter recovery time. Studies have shown in other species that HBOT increases circulating, pluri-potent stem cells from the bone marrow. This effect appears to be mediated by the increase in ostecoclastic activity after HBOT which in turn is part of the mechanism for stem release.

The use of HBOT in the treatment of exercise induced pulmonary hemorrhage (EIPH) shows great promise. There have been reports that range from a permanent elimination of signs to no effect. The exact mechanism for the effect of HBOT in EIPH is yet to be determined.

Hyperbaric Oxygen Therapy and Blood Loss

In acute blood loss due to hemorrhage or RBC destruction the maintenance of adequate organ function and viability depends on an adequate supply of oxygen to cover consumption by the tissues. In the normal patient the majority of oxygen is transported to the tissues attached to hemoglobin with a small amount dissolved in the plasma. With the loss of red cells the oxygen capacity may be significantly reduced. Hemorrhage and RBC destruction may produce a loss of red cells significantly reducing the oxygen capacity. Hyperbaric oxygen therapy can increase the dissolved oxygen concentration to a level that will sustain organ function and viability. At 3 ATA the dissolved oxygen can reach a level of approximately 6.38 volumes %. This level has been shown in humans to provide adequate oxygen for the brain.

Hyperbaric therapy may have an application in RBC loss for; 1) support of vital functions prior to red cell replacement, 2) sustaining life when replacement is not an option, 3) support in autoimmune hemolytic anemias. In acute hemorrhagic shock, HBOT in conjunction with volume replacement may be life saving or supportive prior to blood replacement. In autoimmune hemolytic disease transfusions may be in-effective or contraindicated and HBOT may support body functions until the immune mediated component is under control.

Hyperbaric Oxygen Therapy and Carbon Monoxide Toxicity

HBOT may be indicated for animals that have suffered carbon monoxide (CO) inhalation such as may occur from smoke or exhaust inhalation resulting from combustion of carbon fuel sources. Carbon monoxide toxicity results from a chain of events that begin with a 200 fold increase in affinity of hemoglobin for CO over oxygen. Oxygen cannot bind to hemoglobin; there is a left shift in the oxyhemoglobin dissociation curve and eventually respiratory depression. These events result in cellular oxygen deprivation and organ compromise. Carbon monoxide may also bind to some extravascular proteins such as cytochrome oxidases, increase the level of nitric oxide and promote oxidative stress. In both laboratory animal and human studies, HBOT has been shown have a better outcome in patients than the administration of oxygen at surface pressure. The mechanisms by which HBOT provides a benefit include; the significant increase in oxygen levels decreases the CO half life and increases dissociation of CO from hemoglobin, dissociation of CO from cytochrome oxidases, and the prevention of oxidative injury by decreasing leukocyte adherence to vascular endothelium. The administration of 100% oxygen at pressures between 2.5-3 ATA has been shown to be beneficial in animal models and human clinical studies. Horses and other species with smoke inhalation and respiratory distress from involvement in barn and house fires will benefit from HBOT.

Hyperbaric Oxygen Therapy Protocols

Oxygen, as most drugs, has a dose (ATA/over time), frequency, and duration of treatment profile. Research into the application of HBOT in humans has provided some animal protocols, but virtually there are no specific equine protocols that have been derived from controlled research. Most equine and some small animal protocols have either been derived from trial and error in clinical practice or developed by extrapolation from human protocols. Treatment regiments, for the most part, apply oxygen in the 2-3 ATA range. Greater than 3 ATA should not be employed as this greatly increases the risk of oxygen toxicity. Two philosophies exist on treatment times; 1) a lower pressure (1.5-2.0 ATA) for a longer time, 2) higher pressure (2.0-3.0 ATA) for a shorter time. Many protocols currently being used in the horse have a 45-60 minute treatment time at 2-3 ATA. The frequency of treatment and the number of treatments will depend on the nature of the problem being treated. At this point we have no controlled research data in the horse to verify specific dose, frequency, and duration other than those developed through clinical experiences. For example, in the case of a compromised, non-healing wound the treatment protocol used might include 45-60 minutes in the chamber, breathing 100% oxygen at a pressure of 2.5 ATA every other day. The wound progress would be monitored and treatment would continue until the wound healed or until healing was significantly improved. This could require as little as ten treatments or as many as 30 treatments depending on wound size and reasons for lack of healing (infection, loss of blood supply etc.). The frequency of every other day allows periods of low oxygen tensions to occur in the wound which is necessary for stiumulation of angiogenesis. For the prevention of potential laminitis in a patient with a retained placenta or other causes a course of therapy might be 45-60 minutes in the chamber breathing 100% oxygen at a pressure of 2.5 ATA once or twice daily for 3-5 days. We have also successfully prevented progression of very early laminitis signs in some cases with 100% oxygen at 2.5 ATA daily for 3-5 days. Patients that may require long term therapy would include osteomyelitis, severe septic arthritis, severely compromised wounds, intracranial and abdominal abscesses, and peripheral neuropathies.

Hyperbaric Oxygen Chambers and Operation

In the United States hyperbaric oxygen chambers are classified by the National Fire Protection Agency (NFPA) into chambers for human occupancy (Classes A & B) and those for animal occupancy but no human occupancy (Class C). Regulations for construction and operation differ depending on the chamber class. Class A human multiplace chambers are usually pressurized using air while the patient breaths 100% oxygen by mask. Class B human single occupancy chambers are usually pressurized with 100% oxygen. There are equine chambers available that pressurize with either 100% oxygen or air (mask 100% oxygen). It is important to note that regulations for Class C chambers specifically state, **no human occupancy**.

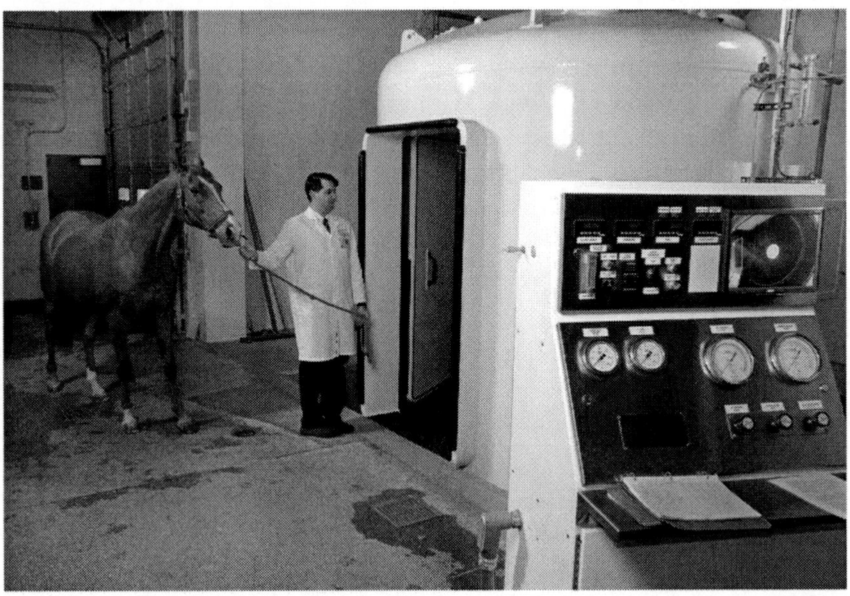

Figure 10. State of the art vertical large animal hyperbaric chamber.

Hyperbaric chambers should be constructed to meet standards and guidelines of pressure vessel inspection and certification agencies. This includes use of appropriate materials, proper construction, and appropriate pressure testing. Size of the chamber will depend on the species being treated. Chambers are available for animals that can be used with mice and other laboratory animals to the equine species. In some venues human monoplace chambers are being used for small animal therapy.

Basic characteristics of animal hyperbaric chambers should include consideration of the comfort of the patient; visibility of the patient by outside attendants; appropriate grounding of the patient; elimination of any ignition sources inside of the chamber; emergency access, ability to monitor chamber pressure, temperature, humidity, time and percent oxygen; accurate, reliable, user friendly control module; ease of cleaning and disinfection; externally environmentally controlled chamber location (Figure 10).

Patient and operator safety is paramount in any hyperbaric program and chamber operation. Proper chamber operation is achieved with proper training in the theory and practice of hyperbaric medicine and the development of protocols addressing continuous training of personnel in operation, safety, and maintenance of the chamber. It is highly recommended that a qualified, hyperbaric safety officer be on staff to monitor chamber operations and to help develop safety protocols and risk assessment procedures.

Conclusion

Hyperbaric oxygen therapy has been employed as a complimentary and primary therapy in human medicine for many years. Hyperbaric therapy in veterinary medicine has been practiced for several years but lacks basic, controlled research information in the various species. There is a wealth of anecdotal, case based information as well as some research information in small animals, pigs and laboratory animals that have contributed to the development of the successful HBOT use in veterinary medicine. Treatment protocols and indications have been extrapolated from this information for animal hyperbaric therapy. The case based information is extremely encouraging. Hyperbaric therapy should always be considered and offered as another weapon in the veterinarian's arsenal of therapies because of its ability to improve healing, provide for tissue salvage, aid in infection control, and reduce edema and inflammation.

Suggested Reading

Bennett PB, Elliott DH. *The Physiology and medicine of diving*. 4th ed. London: Philadelphia; 1993.

Kindwall EP, Whelan HT. *Hyperbaric medicine practice*. 3rd ed. Flagstaff, AZ: Best Pub. Co.; 2008.

Sheffield PJ, Smith APS. *Physiological and Pharmacological Basis of Hyperbaric Oxygen Therapy*. Flagstaff, AZ: Best Pub. Co.; 2002.

In: Rehabilitating the Athletic Horse
Editors: H. W. Jann et al., pp. 87-115
ISBN: 978-1-678-1-60876-672-7

Chapter 6

EQUINE INTRA-ARTICULAR INJECTION

***Bradford G. Bentz*[1] *and Mark S. Revenaugh*[2]**
[1]VMD, MS, DACVIM, ACVP (Equine), Hagyard Equine Medical Institute in Lexington, Kentucky, USA
[2]DVM. Northwest Equine Performance LLC, Mulino, OR, USA

ABSTRACT

Within the last 25 years, the administration of medications directly into a joint has evolved into a skill and a mandatory procedure that nearly any equine veterinarian is expected to perform. The procedure has become an invaluable tool for the diagnosis, treatment and maintenance of joint health in horses used for any type of athletic use. . The ever- increasing demands on such performance horses has produced a boon in our understanding of the pathophysiology of joint disorders in horses. As a result, we have seen an ever-increasing improvement in the specificity of therapy, and an increasing focus on joint health maintenance with Disease Modifiying Osteoarthritis Drugs (DMOAD), systemic medications and complementary therapies.

INTRODUCTION

Among veterinarians who engage in significant sport and race horse practice, the utilization of intra-articular injection and therapy has become essential in order to continue to offer these athletes the ability to continue to exercise, train and compete in comfort and to their athletic potential, while also modifying the progression of any joint pathology. Given these benefits however, there is also a potential for inappropriate use and over-utilization of these techniques. As such, there is a fine, yet indistinct line, that every veterinarian must define for him/herself in order to utilize intra-articular injection and therapy in a responsible manner that is of benefit to the horse and to the individuals involved with the preparation, training and competition of that animal. This line is not always easy to define given the numerous influences and pressures on a veterinarian involved with treating and managing horses that exercise, train and compete. At certain higher levels of competition, the veterinarian is often faced with the difficulty of managing and diagnosing horses that are not overtly lame or that are experiencing poorly defined deterioration in their levels of performance.

The purpose of this chapter is to outline the basic information and current understandings of intra-articular injection and therapeutic techniques in order to facilitate successful management of such horses with beneficial and responsible practice techniques.

JOINT INFLAMMATION AND OSTOEARTHRITIS

It is not within the scope of this chapter to specifically outline and review inflammatory arthropathies. However, a very brief description will be helpful to frame a later discussion of the various intra-articular therapies available to the practitioner. There is increasing interest in intervening in joint disorders earlier than by the time osteoarthritis has become apparent. A single traumatic event, such as an osteochondral chip fracture, may produce an acute form of arthropathy. If these acute traumatic events are not managed acutely and intensively (e.g. fragment removal), many of these acute traumas will produce chronic and often severe osteoarthritis. Frequently, once the acute joint trauma is initially managed, continued long-term management is often necessary to facilitate joint health and to control the progression of joint osteoarthritis. However, most horses probably develop the chronic form of osteoarthritis as a result of repetitive mild joint trauma from years of exercise, training and athletic competition. This chronic form is often insidious, with initial capsulitis and synovitis progressing to overt osteoarthritis if untreated. Although poor conformation is likely to be a predisposing factor, horses with excellent conformation also develop capsulitis and synovitis from today's rigorous training and competition schedules. Capsulitis and synovitis are believed to result in a cascade of inflammatory mediators (initiated by interleukin-1) that can lead to the release of various enzymes associated with cartilage degeneration, including collagenase, stromolysin, serine proteinases, matrix metalloproteinase and others. This enzymatic degradation is the major factor that leads to development of advanced osteoarthritis. The results are articular cartilage damage, synovial membrane thickening, and joint capsule fibrosis. Osteoarthritis is a byproduct of the wear and tear and daily trauma beginning with enzymatic release, followed by cartilage degradation, leaching of proteoglycan and unwinding of the collagen due to the inflammatory mediators. Collagen molecules then appear to stimulate more inflammation, and a vicious cycle is initiated. Because of this, some of the most promising techniques to control and manage this disease process include early intervention at the capsulitis and synovitis stages, and the utilization of chondroprotective or disease-modifying osteoarthritic drugs (DMOADs). We are certainly becoming increasingly more focused on the role of synovitis and the enzymatic degradation that occurs in the joint as precursors to the development of OA for horses with the more common chronic, repetitive trauma-induced arthropathies.

Subchondral bone injury can also occur as a result of a single episode or repetitive overuseage. These injuries often appear the same as joint injury, despite the fact that the primary injury is proximal or distal to the joint surface. Treatment of such injuries with intraarticular therapies is generally unrewarding. Similarly, response to intra-articular anesthesia is variable.

Osteoarthritis as a result of "joint instability" is often overlooked as an underlying cause of joint pathology. Diarthoidial joints rely upon soft-tissue structures for joint stability. Examples include collateral ligaments, tendons, menisci, cruciate ligaments, muscle groups as well as the joint capsule. If the joint is not stable, abnormal joint motion may result. Secondary inflammation occurs as the joint is challenged an abnormal range of motion is experienced. Resulting nonspecific symptoms of joint- inflammation may then occur (swelling, heat, effusion, pain etc.). If such a joint is injected, it will likely experience profound temporary improvement. However, if the instability/ mechanical issue is not addressed, the inflammation is likely to return when the joint stability is challenged again.

In summary, osteoarthritis is a disease process. In its mild (early) form, OA occurs as a physiologic proccss. Ovcr timc, thc physiologic process of a chronic unhealthy synovial environment can lead to structural and even mechanical issues, (loss of joint capsule elasticity, and/or radiographic changes associated with oa etc.).

Mechanisms for the Control of Joint Inflammation

It is probably inescapable that horses that are in prolonged regular training, competition or other exercise will develop some form of joint pathology. Recognizing the early signs of joint inflammation is important in reducing long-term effects and the development of osteoarthritis. Early appropriate intervention to control joint inflammation is more likely to facilitate joint health and performance longevity at the expected level. Control of joint inflammation is not restricted to intra-articular interventions. Non-articular therapeutic options for joint inflammation are reviewed in another chapter in this book. Generally speaking, these options are either utilized before intra-articular therapy is instituted, or they are used in conjunction with intra-articular therapies for management and control of joint inflammation and osteoarthritis. Rest, cooling therapy and controlled exercise are probably the most ubiquitously utilized management strategies for lameness in horses. However, once OA is in its later stages, rest may actually exacerbate the clinical symptoms associated with joint pain. Furthermore, trainers and riders oftentimes have tremendous pressures to continue competing despite joint pain. It is the author's experience that a horse who has experienced an acute "one time" trauma or soft tissue injury will benefit most from the rest time.

These strategies are used alone or in conjunction with other therapies, but their importance in management of lameness cannot be overstated. Intravenous, intramuscular and oral joint therapies are widely available and appear to have a definite place in management of joint inflammation and control of the progression of osteoarthritis. Judicious anti-inflammatory therapy is a powerful tool to control joint inflammation and includes systemic (oral, IM and IV), topical and intra-articular therapies. Appropriate utilization of these therapies is associated with excellent clinical results and greatly facilitates the control of the progression of joint disease. Frequently, various combinations of therapy from all of the categories are utilized in order to produce excellent clinical results with the greatest duration of efficacy and benefit to joint health.

Medications Utilized for Intra-Articular Injection

Mepivacaine (Carbocaine)

Mepivicaine is almost exclusively used for diagnostic local anesthesia of equine joints. This drug exhibits medium duration of action (similar to lidocaine), rapid onset of action, and analgesia appears to begin to subside between 1 and 2 hours after blocking. It is reported to be twice as potent as lidocaine. Its potency, moderate duration of action and reportedly reduced level of joint irritation (relative to lidocaine) may explain its ubiquitous use as the local anesthetic of choice for diagnostic blocks of the equine joint. Frequently, following diagnostic anesthesia of a joint, a therapeutic intra-articular intervention is desired. Traditionally, it has been considered less than optimal to treat a joint on the same day that the joint has been anesthetized. This presumption has not been substantiated. Furthermore, some horses have been observed to be less lame the day after a joint has been "blocked". It has been speculated that in such instances, cases the carbocaine may exhibit some anti-inflammatory properties. The dosage of carbocaine varies for intrarticular use. Most joints are adequately anesthetized with 4 ml of carbocaine. The larger joints may require substantially larger volumes of carbocaine to achieve complete anesthesia.

Morphine

Morphine is an opoid narcotic of producing significant analgesia. It is most often used in horses either by systemic (VI or IM) or by epidural administration for intense analgesia in the horse. However, this medication may also be utilized for local analgesia in horses experiencing severe joint pain. Morphine would be administered intra-articular injection for this effect. However, the dose, safety and efficacy of this use has not yet been reported.

Hyaluronic Acid (HA)

Hyaluronic acid (also called Hyaluronan or hyaluronate) is a non-sulfated glycosaminoglycan distributed widely throughout connective, epithelial, and neural tissues. It is one of the chief components of the extracellular matrix, and is a major component of the synovial fluid, increasing the viscosity of the fluid. Along with lubricin, it is one of the synovial fluid's main lubricating components. Hyaluronic acid (HA) is an important component of articular cartilage, where it is present as a coat around each chondrocyte.

When aggrecan monomers bind to hyaluronan in the presence of link protein, large highly negatively-charged aggregates form. These aggregates imbibe water and are responsible for the resilience of cartilage (its resistance to compression). HA is harvested from such sources as rooster comb, umbilical cord, etc. and formulated for intra-articular injection. HA appears to help restore the function of the naturally occurring hyaluronic acid within the joint to improve the lubrication and stimulate natural production of HA. HA is often used in conjunction with steroids. Oral forms of HA are also available and are covered in another chapter in this book.

Table 1.

Trade Name	Manufacturer	Molecular Weight (Daltons) *	Concentration	Recommended Dose †
Equron	Solvay Animal Health	$1.5\text{-}2.0 \times 10^6$	5 mg/mL	10 mg
Equiflex	Chesapeake Biological	1.0×10^6	5 mg/mL	10 mg
HY 50	Bexo Pharma		17 mg/mL	51 mg
Hyalovet (Hyalovet-20)	Fort Dodge/ Vetrepharm	$4\text{-}7 \times 10^5$	10 mg/mL	20 mg
Hycoat ‡	Neogen	$>1.0 \times 10^6$	5 mg/mL	30 mg
Hylartin V (Hylartil Vet)	Pharmacia and Upjohn	3.5×10^6	10 mg/mL	20 mg
Hyvisc	Vetmedica	2.1×10^6	11 mg/mL	20 mg
Legend (Hyonate)	Bayer Corporation	3.0×10^5	10 mg/mL	40 mg
MAP-5§	Vetrepharm	7.5×10^5	10.3 mg/mL (2ml) 5 mg/ml (10ml)	20 mg
Synacid	Schering-Plough	$0.15\text{-}0.20 \times 10^6$	10 mg/mL	50 mg

* As stated by manufacturer

† Intra-articular dosages are those recommended for small-medium-sized joints (eg, metacarpophalangeal). Some manufacturers recommend twice the dose for larger joints (eg, tibiotarsal).

‡ Marketed as an ophthalmic preparation, but popular for intra-articular use at this dose.

§ Marketed as a topical preparation for wounds, but used intra-articularly.

Hyaluronic acid has been reported to exhibit anti-inflammatory effects, pain relief and improvement of joint mobility. Analgesic properties of this compound are believed to be due to reduction in the sensitivity of articular nerve endings and anti-inflammatory effects. Disease modifying effects of HA are postulated but are not yet characterized. Hyaluronic acid has been demonstrated to regulate PGE_2 synthesis and to scavenge oxygen-derived free radicals and degradative enzymes. Hyaluronic acid is proposed to potentiate the synthesis of Hyaluronic acid by synovial cells and to promote proteoglycan synthesis. HA is reported to protect cartilage from the effects of IL-1 and inflammatory mediators. Cartilage sparing effects of HA are reported to occur following intra-articular injection of HA by suppression of inflammatory cytokines and degradative proteinases.

The most commonly used HA products are Hylartin-V, HyVisc, Legend or Hyalovet. These products are labeled for intra-articular use, insuring product purity and consistency. MAP-5 is hyaluronic acid used in sperm extender and is not labeled for, but has been used extensively in equine joint therapy. Although anecdotal reports of use of this product have suggested good clinical response, safety and comparative clinical efficacy to the products labeled for equine intra-articular injection has not been reported.

Low Versus High Molecular Weight HA

Experimental evidence, has suggested that using the highest molecular weight (thickness) of HA provides the most benefit. It has been suggested that Hyaluronic acid with molecular weight exceeding 1 $X10^6$d performs superiorly to lower molecular weight preparations, but this claim is not universally supported. Cartilage sparing effects of higher molecular weight preparations appear to be superior to lower molecular weight preparations in some models. However, the translation into biologic, in vivo protection is less clear. Better clinical results have been reported in human and equine trials utilizing higher molecular weight compounds, but these findings are not universally supported in various research models of synovial inflammation and joint disease.

Disease-Modifying Effects of Hyaluronan Relative to Molecular Weight

Cell/Tissue	Effect	Influence of MW (Daltons)	Comments
Leukocytes	↓ migration, chemotaxis, adhesion	$>1 \times 10^6$ superior to $< 1 \times 10^6$	
	↓ free radical scavenging	$>1 \times 10^6$ superior to $< 1 \times 10^6$	
Synovial fibroblasts (B cells)	↑synthesis of HA	0.5×10^6 optimal	High concentrations of low MW ↓synthesis as does MW $> 3\text{-}4 \times 10^6$
	↓PGE2 release	2×10^6 superior to $0.2\text{-}1.0 \times 10^6$	
Chondrocytes/ cartilage	↓PGE2 release	2×10^6 superior to 0.5×10^6	
	↓Proteoglycan release	$0.3 \times 10^6 = 2 \times 10^6$	
	↑PG synthesis	0.8×10^6 superior to $<0.3 \times 10^6$	Low MW inhibits synthesis
	↓IL-1 induced, ↓PG and collagen synthesis	1×10^6 superior to $<0.5 \times 10^6$	
	↓Chondrocyte apoptosis	$0.5\text{-}0.7 \times 10^6$ superior to $<0.1 \times 10^6$	1×10^6 less effective than $0.5\text{-}0.7 \times 10^6$
	↑TIMP-1 release (Tissue Inhibitor of Metallopreoteinase)	2×10^6 superior to 1×10^6 superior to 0.5×10^6	

The ideal molecular weight of HA for clinical use remains unclear. One recommendation is for the use of HA with molecular weight in the range of 0.5 to 2.0 X 10^6d. Despite the apparent trend to select for high molecular weight HA, there appears to be some evidence that molecular weights greater than 3-4 x 10^6d may lead to reduction of endogenous HA production, as is found with the use of low molecular weight HA. Thus, the recommended range for optimal HA molecular weight may be partially dependent on the criteria used to evaluate its effects. (see above table).

Combination Therapy with Corticosteroid and Hyaluronic Acid

The use of a combination of a corticosteroid with hyaluronic acid for intra-articular therapy is standard practice in equine medicine. A lower dose of steroid is believed to be facilitated by the concurrent administration of HA. Furthermore, the cartilage sparing effect of HA is also potentially a benefit in this combination therapy. Corticosteroid and HA combination therapy has been reported to be synergistic in human patients with osteoarthritis. Additionally, variables associated with commercial product formulations including cost of the HA product, or the size and type of syringe may need to be considered in the selection of the formulations utilized. Ultimately, the choice of which HA product to use is made largely on the veterinarian's personal experiences. Traditionally, high molecular weight products have been considered to be superior. At this time, anecdotal evidence does not necessarily support this finding.

Polysulfated Glysosaminoglycan (PSGAG)

Polysulfated glycosaminoglycan (PSGAG) is a semi-synthetic preparation from bovine trachea that is comprised principally of chondroitin sulfate, a glycosaminoglycan found in the aggregated proteoglycan of cartilage. The use of this compound is associated with reports of improved clinical signs in both human and equine patients. PSGAG is purported to have both chondroprotective and anti-inflammatory properties; however, the exact nature and mechanism(s) by which it exerts these effects are unknown. Used in humans since the 1960s, PSGAG administration leads to reductions in the severity of clinical signs in human and equine arthritis patients. Clinical improvement is likely attributable to anti-inflammatory effects, including the inhibition of PGE2 synthesis and of cytokine release. Early reports suggested that PSGAG stimulates the synthesis of proteoglycans and collagen by chondrocytes, an effect that appeared to contribute to the healing of damaged cartilage. Subsequent studies have failed to demonstrate any stimulation of proteoglycan synthesis, and it is currently accepted that the stimulation of cartilage repair is not among the central mechanisms of PSGAG action. While PSGAG is considered by many to be an effective means of preventing cartilage degeneration in a joint, it does not appear to heal joint defects. The continued investigation of this compound has failed to show significant effects in the early healing of cartilage lesions. In fact, repair tissue in healing cartilage under the influence of this compound appeared to be inferior to that found in untreated animals. Instead, PSGAG is believed to help prevent cartilage degeneration. PSGAG works on the collagen fibers and intercollagenous tissues that comprise the matrix, or origination point, of joint cartilage. PSGAG has anticatabolic effects; it is capable of inhibiting the activity of a number of degradative enzymes known to be present in articular tissues. Various animal arthritis models have provided support for a disease-modifying effect of PSGAG *in vivo* and, in most cases, beneficial effects were primarily attributed to the inhibition of degradative enzymes. Despite these findings, some clinicians do not believe that the drug can even protect cartilage. This alternative viewpoint has been substantiated by other studies that have shown PSGAG to have little beneficial effect on cartilage degeneration.

PSGAG can be administered intra-articularly or intramuscularly. However, intra-articular administration of PSGAG has been associated with an increased incidence of joint infection and with a sterile synovitis (joint flare) at a rate that was reported to exceed that seen from corticosteroid intra-articular injection. A related study appeared to show that using an antibiotic in conjunction with the PSGAG prevented infection (amikacin 125 mg). These findings have reduced the apparent clinical administration of PSGAG intra-articularly and many veterinarians now opt for the less problematic intramuscular version of Adequan. Because of the reported association of intra-articular PSGAG use and sepsis, it is important to follow proper aseptic technique and include amikacin while using IA adequan. From 1999-2008, Luitpold has had 3 reports of adverse reactions to IA Adequan (.00002% of all doses sold). (personal communication; Allyn Mann). While it is likely to be safer, it is probable that intramuscular Adequan produces reduced clinical benefit in comparison to intra-articular Adequan. The frequency of PSGAG administration is usually based on the therapeutic response and its duration. There is considerable variability in the symptomatic relief with PSGAG treatment; typically, when a favorable therapeutic response occurs, it appears to frequently be rapid. Adequan is the best-known PSGAG product; others include Cartophen (pentosan polysulfate) and Rumalon (glycosaminoglycan peptide complex). Cartophen and Rumalon are not licensed in the United States.

Intra articular adequan was used routinely by equine practitioners from the late 1980's thru the early 1990's. As increased risk of joint flare and sepsis was identified, its use as an intra- articular medication was virtually halted, despite strong evidence supporting its beneficial effects. Specifically, following IA Adequan, the injected joint appeared to exhibit increased susceptibilty to stapylococcal infections. Presumably, the decrease use of IA adequan was because equine veterinarians were trying to avoid the problems associated with post injection flare or sepsis, (loss of client confidence as well as possible legal ramifications).

Over recent years, use of intra-articular Adequan has become a routine-practice again with many equine veterinarians. Many practitioners choose to add steroid to the IA adequan in a fashion similar to use of steroid and HA. Some practitioners claim superior results with intra-articular Adequan vs intra-articular HA presumably due to the cartilage sparing effect. These reports are anecdotal. Definitive studies comparing use of HA and Adequan are lacking.

Interleukin-1 Receptor Antagonist Protein (IRAP)

Interleukin-1 receptor protein antagonist (IRAP) is a therapeutic agent recently introduced into the arsenal of intra-articular therapies. As its name implies, this protein works by binding to interleukin-1, preventing it from binding to the Interleukin-1 (IL-1) receptor.

IL-1, through its receptor, is the major progenitor in the inflammatory cascade that leads to synovitis and joint pain. By blocking this interaction it is believed that pain and inflammation in the joint can be moderated or eliminated. The result of this would be the facilitation of joint health and healing. This therapy has been reported to be helpful for arthritis and back pain in human patients. It requires a series of intra-articular injections. Preparation of the injected product involves a protocol for autologous harvest of the antagonist protein from the pateint's blood. This procedure has now been adapted for use in equine joints.

The commercially available human product, called Orthokine, consists of a packet for harvesting the protein from the whole blood. This product is utilized similarly for autologous harvest of the protein from whole horse blood. The process for obtaining IRAP is relatively easy but requires additional spccific cquipment, such as a centrifuge that accommodates 60 ml syringes and an incubator. The orthokine kit provides a 60 ml syringe containing glass beads to stimulate monocytic production of the antagonist protein and anticoagulant. A jugular vein is aseptically prepared and 60 ml of blood is harvested. The syringes are then incubated at 37 degrees C for 24 hours (+ 5 hours). The syringes are then centrifuged to separate IRAP rich plasma from the blood. The plasma is then harvested in 4 ml aliquots in a 6 ml syringe and frozen until use. Prior to injecting into a joint, the IRAP plasma is passed through a 0.2 micro millipore filter. Typically 4 ml is injected once a week for 3 treatments. In large volume joints such as the stifle, the investigators of this product in horses have used an 8 ml dose. Depending on the condition being treated, the investigators have rested the recipient horses until they receive the second injection. They are then permitted to go back to training. One study protocol utilized as series of 3 injections of the affected joint. Associated articular soft tissue injuries are important to consider in treating any lameness. Therefore, as with other intra-articular therapies, response to treatment is likely to be incomplete or of short duration if such an injury exists. Joints affected with synovitis or mild degenerative joint disease are reported to have responded best to this therapy.

Despite the promising reports from the investigators, not all clinicians are in agreement with the efficacy of IRAP therapy. Much of these differing opinions may be a result of differing criteria for case selection. IRAP exhibits characteristics of a Disease Modifying Osteoarthritis Drug (DMOAD). As such, it has been suggested to be helpful as a long-term disease-modifying agent to reduce and delay the return of inflammation following intra-articularcorticosteriods and hyaluronic acid treatment. This approach was suggested to help minimize need to repeat joint injections with hyaluronic acid and corticosteroids. IRAP has also been recommended for joints that have been treated with intra-articular corticosteroids, but are either unresponsive or have become unresponsive. IRAP has been utilized as initial therapy for many horses. However, because of the significant expense of the procedure, this approach will not be universally feasible for all horses and in all types of equine practices. Because corticosteroids are much less expensive to utilize, effective and also exhibit disease modifying characteristics, they are probably an excellent initial approach for many or most initial therapies. IRAP is available if and when corticosteroids fail to produce the desired result when the owner is willing to undertake the financial commitment of this therapy. Another likely application of IRAP may include intra-articular therapy for a horse with an upcoming competition and that cannot have corticosteroid (or other medication) in a drug test. In fact, IRAP has been utilized in some horses with recurring joint problems that have an upcoming major event, in order to avoid glucocorticoid use. This approach reported to be effective in managing these chronic joint problems and to facilitate competition in the targeted competition possibly without perpetuation cartilage damage.

Despite these apparent benefits, IRAP therapy requires a series of joint injections and the responses to the therapy have been variable, and at least partly dependent on the joint pathology. These factors may limit IRAP as a viable and effective treatment for impending competition. Additionally, care should be taken to closely control the environment of the samples so as to avoid production of unwanted stress proteins in the IRAP "Broth". Specifically, temperature fluctuations should be avoided while handling the whole blood preparation. It should be emphasized that at the time of writing this chapter, identification and quantification of equine IRAP in the IRAP-sample has not been achieved. We are presuming its presence and hoping that some additional non specific growth factors may present. A newer product called IRAP 2 is currently available. The related product in human medicine reportedly produces significantly more IRAP protein.

CORTICOSTEROIDS

The Steroid Stigma

Corticosteroids, as a class of drugs, have received much negative attention in the past two decades. This attention has severely skewed many owners, trainers, riders and some veterinarians to the point of becoming insistent on the strict avoidance of the administration of steroids in any manner. As performance horse and sport horse veterinarians, we have surely encountered the situation in which we wish to utilize steroid therapy in order to achieve the result the trainer and owner are demanding. However, these same clients may concurrently demand that steroids not be used. In these instances, it may be necessary to attempt other therapy, such as IRAP, but it is also important to address the potential for a less than ideal response to the alternative therapy. Corticosteroids became blamed for complications related to their use in racehorses with arthritis, that sustained injury of the treated joint following their use. Unfortunately, it is not the drug class that is responsible for this occurrence, but rather the inappropriate selection of the clinical situation in which they were utilized. Adding to the already damaged image of corticosteroid use in the horse, a body of research was produced that suggested that the use of corticosteroids in joints was associated with cartilaginous damage. An association of corticosteroid use with laminitis has also become common. These factors have further fueled the apprehension of intra-articular corticosteroid use in the horse.

The realities of appropriate intra-articular corticosteroid use are dramatically different than these perceptions. As veterinarians, we have a responsibility to educate and communicate these realities to our clients, and to the equine industry as a whole. The damage created by steroid injections was primarily in horses with end-stage osteoarthritis, where the disease progresses even in the face of treatment. IA steroids may also "mask" a joint injury or a soft tissue injury which would be best treated with rest or other therapies. Substantiation for a direct link between corticosteroid administration and arthritis remains unproven by numerous investigations. Recent studies have suggested no difference in cartilage lesions of horses that had surgery and corticosteroid injections when compared to their controls. The current conclusion of involved researchers, clinicians and practitioners is that intra-articular corticosteroids may potentially aggravate existing cartilage lesions in horses involved in intense exercise, but this occurrence is less prevalent than previously believed and less than what public perception suggests. Indeed, most of the problems associated with intra-articular corticosteroid administration can be attributed to poor injection technique (infection) or poor selection of corticosteroid doses and products. Despite these findings, exceptionally high doses of corticosteroids and/or frequent repetitive utilization of corticosteroids in the same joint are interventions that should be critically evaluated and avoided by attending veterinarians. The need to intervene with repetitive intra-articular corticosteroid therapy should strongly indicate the need for further diagnostic evaluation and consideration of other possible complicating problems of the affected joint or the presence of advanced disease. Further diagnostic workup is reportedly indicated if a horse requires re-injection within two months of treatment. Added caution is warranted with injection frequency in high-motion joints (e.g. fetlock and coffin joints). At least a six-month window between treatments was suggested to be prudent with a need for more frequent injections potentially indicating undiagnosed problems.

Current research has proven that when used correctly, corticosteroids are very effective and relatively inexpensive medications in the intervention and control of joint disease. They can be included in the class of medications considered to be "disease modifying" medications. The enzymes that are produced by diseased or inflamed joints are responsible for the damage to normal cartilage. Joints that are inflamed must be treated with anti-inflammatory medication (often with hyaluronic acid) in order to curtail the production and release of these damaging enzymes and to re-establish the production of normal joint fluid. Because inflamed joint tissues will not produce normal, thick, adequately lubricating hyaluronic acid and joint fluid, intra-articular corticosteroids are important for the re-establishment of the ability of the joint to produce healthy hyaluronic acid. Clinical signs of joint disease such as lameness, synovial effusion, heat and pain on joint flexion can usually be reduced more quickly and for a longer duration when intra-articular corticosteroids are utilized in comparison to most other intra-articular monotherapies.

Corticosteroid Mechanisms and Duration of Action

Disease modifying properties of corticosteroids have been proposed. The two major mediators of cartilage degeneration include interleukin-1 and tumor necrosis factor α. These two mediators are suppressed by the effects of corticosteroids. Corticosteroids are also believed to inhibit the movement of inflammatory cells into the site of inflammation and inhibit neutrophil function by impairing release of lysosomal enzymes and neutrophil phagocytosis. Corticosteroids inhibit prostaglandin production primarily through the inhibition of phospholipase A2 through the steroid-inducible group of proteins known as lipocortins. Inhibition of phospholipase A2 prevents the breakdown of membrane phospholipids to fatty acids, which are subsequently oxygenated by the cyclooxygenase and lipoxygenase pathways into inflammatory eicosanoids. In contrast to non-steroidal anti-inflammatory drugs that only inhibit the cyclooxygenase pathway, corticosteroids inhibit both eicosanoid pathways. They are therefore comparatively more effective anti-inflammatory agents. Other less well-defined anti-inflammatory actions of corticosteroids include inhibition of metalloproteinases, inhibition of monocyte-macrophage complexes at the site of inflammation, inhibition of chemotaxis and adherence of neutrophils to the vascular endothelium, and inhibition of plasminogen activator activity. The inhibition of cytokines and degradative enzymes involved in the pathogenesis of osteoarthritis is the probable mechanism for the exhibition of DMOAD characteristics by corticosteroids. Studies have demonstrated these effects at low doses are capable of producing cartilage sparing effects without affecting the chondrocyte.

Estimating the duration of action and the relative potency of intra-articular corticosteroids is difficult. It has been suggested that the duration of action is directly related to the lipid solubility of the corticosteroid. However, the duration of action is not necessarily determined by the continued presence of the drug in the joint fluid. Concentrations of methylprednisolone and triamcinolone can only be detected in synovial fluid for a short period of time following injection, but the clinical anti-inflammatory effects are reported to last much longer. Additionally, corticosteroids are prodrugs and must be hydrolyzed into their active forms. The rate of hydrolysis within a joint may affect both the onset and duration of action, and the potency of the drug. However, the rate of drug hydrolysis may not be that important since most corticosteroids are rapidly converted to their active forms within synovial fluid. Although there are many caveats in determining duration of action and potency of IA corticosteroids, it is generally considered that methylprednisolone and betamethasone have an intermediate to long duration of action and triamcinolone has an intermediate duration of action. Regarding potency, it has been estimated that betamethasone is more potent than tiamcinolone, which is more potent than methylprednisolone. However, not all veterinarians are in agreement with these generalizations. (see table comparing published duration and potency of corticosteroids).

Triamcinolone Acetonide (Vetalog, Kenalog)

Triamcinolone is reported to exhibit approximately five times the anti-inflammatory potency of cortisol and up to 1.25 times the potency of prednisolone. Studies have demonstrated favorable effects of triamcinolone on the degree of clinically detectable lameness, and on synovial fluid, synovial membrane, and articular cartilage morphological parameters compared to placebo treatment. This is in contrast to the detrimental effects on articular cartilage that were found with methylprednisolone using the same experimental model. This finding has served as the basis for the selection of triamcinolone over methylprednisolone in high motion joints and in other clinical situations in which these proposed cartilage sparing effects are desirable. Despite this argument, other *in vitro* investigations have suggested that triamcinolone at all doses is more detrimental to cartilage metabolism than methylprednisolone. However, the general impression of most investigators and equine practitioners is that triamcinolone is probably more supportive of overall cartilage and joint health than the other commonly utilized corticosteroids. Additionally, triamcinolone appears to have a significant regional anti-inflammatory effect. The recommended dose of triamcinolone acetonide from the package insert is 6 to 18 mg per horse. However, few practicing equine veterinarians appear to be comfortable with utilizing this drug beyond a total dose of 18 mg. The reason for this limit is significant anecdotal clinical experience that associates these higher total dosages with the development of acute refractory laminitis in the horse. Also for this reason triamcinolone should be used with caution in horses predisposed to laminitis, (ponies, cushings-like phenotype older horses). The development of laminitis following the use of triamconolone acetonide in horses appears to be significantly more likely than with other intra-articular corticosteroids. The package insert also states that intra-articular injection may produce osseous metaplasia. Despite these apparent characteristics, when used appropriately, corticosteroids, and perhaps particularly triamcinolone can improve the health of the joint by its disease-modifying drug characteristics.

Methylprednisolone Acetate (Depomedrol)

Much of the research on intra-articular corticosteroids in horses has focused on methylprednisolone. This drug is probably the most common corticosteroid used for intra-articular therapy in the horse. Several studies have documented detrimental effects of multiple doses of methylprednisolone acetate. A well recognized body of research indicated negative effects on cartilage metabolism, function and repair in high motion joints (carpus, fetlock, tarsocrural, etc). Another investigation indicated that while the drug appeared to inhibit the repair of osteochondral defects, there were no detrimental effects on the quality of the repair tissue. In this investigation, methylprednisolone was reported to induce synovitis for up to 180 days. This report is in contrast to previous studies, which have demonstrated significant antiinflammatory effects of methylprednisolone within joint tissues. It is generally held that methylprednisolone may produce deleterious effects on articular cartilage and it should be used with this in consideration. The package insert recommends a dose of 120 mg for large joints, with a range from 40 to 240 mg. It also states that the duration of action averages 3–4 weeks and that intra-articular injection may occasionally cause a local inflammatory response (joint flare). Though unsubstantiated, lower doses of methylprednisolone (10- 40 mg/joint) appear to be clinically effective and may be less detrimental to articular cartilage. Generally speaking, practitioners are finding that lower doseages of methylprednisolone appear to be as effective as higher doseages. For example, 20 mg methylprednisolone may be sufficient to achieve clinical effect for even joints with a high range of motion joint. Potential for adverse effects of methylprednisolone are likely to be proportional to dosage. Because of the reported detrimental effects on articular cartilage, many equine practitioners limit the use of methylprednisolone in high motion joints, but use it extensively in the distal tarsal joints and proximal interphalangeal joint.

Additional possible negative effects include immediate “joint flare” following ia methylprednisolone injection (severe pain and lameness immediately following injection). Dystrophic mineralization of soft tissue structures following ia administration of methylprednisolone has been described (tendonsheath, joint capsule, adjacent tendon). Establishing a consistent withdrawl time for methylprednisolone has been historically problematic, particularly for Fédération Equestre Internationale (FEI) drug testing. Duration of presence in blood and urine samples appears to depend largely on doseage utilized. At this time the recommended FEI withdrawl time is 14 days, although for larger doses, this interval may be too short. Practitioners are encouraged to exercise caution regarding FEI withdrawl times when using methylprednisolone and competing under FEI rules. Further research is being conducted to clarify safe withdrawl times. Despite these potential negative aspects, methylprednisolone probably remains the most frequently utilized intra-articular steroid in horses.

Betamethasone Sodium Phosphate/ Betamethasone Acetate (Celestone Soluspan, Betasone)

As with triamconolone, little specific research has been done to evaluate the effects of betamethasone on equine articular tissues. Of the limited evaluations performed, there is reportedly minimal detrimental effect of betamethasone on articular tissue in both rested and exercised horses. It is suggested that betamethasone may be less likely to produce joint flare in comparison to other corticosteroids. Despite that these findings are based on limited evaluation of this drug, these perceptions have led many equine practitioners to utilize betamethasone routinely in high motion joints and for its presumptive cartilage sparing effect. The commonly utilized formulation of betamethasone is a human product and combines a water-soluble form (phosphate-presumably for rapid short-acting effect) together with a more lipid-soluble form (acetate- for a more prolonged effect). There is a wide range of doses recommended depending on the size of the joint but most are between 3 to 12 mg/ joint. These recommendations are for human intra-articular therapy. Many equine veterinarians will use higher doses from 6 to 20 mg/joint, depending on the estimated joint size. Betamethasone is generally considered one of the most potent corticosteroids. It is used widely and licensed for use in humans. Periodically betamethasone is not available for purchase. Betamethasone is produced primarily in 2 form: Celestone, (sodium phosphate) and Celestone Soluspan-(sodium phosphate and sodium acetate). The soluspan form offers a more rapid onset of action as well as a long duration of action. Infrequent occurrence of laminitis following large dose betamethasone in ponies has been reported.

Isoflupredone Acetate (Predef 2X)

Isoflupredone has approximately 17 times the anti-inflammatory potency of cortisol and four times the potency of prednisolone. The usual intrasynovial dose for joint inflammation, tendinitis, or bursitis is 5 to 20 mg or more if treating a large joint. Isoflupredone acetate reportedly exerts an inhibitory influence on the mechanisms and the tissue changes associated with inflammation. Vascular permeability is decreased, exudation diminished, and migration of the inflammatory cells markedly inhibited. This drug is not as frequently utilized for intra-articular therapy in horses. Anecdotal reports of temporary intestinal upset resulting from higher doseages of isoflupredone exist. Combining predef 2X with triamcinolone in the same syringe may result in product precipitation, and is not recommended.

Dexamethasone Sodium Phosphate

Although not used widely, dexamethasone has been used for intra-articular administration. It has a rapid onset of action and short duration of action. Corresponding drug withdrawl time is short. At this time, dexamethasone is not used widely for intra-articular use in horses. A form of dexamethasone in an oil base ("Lipotalon") has been available in Europe for intra-articular administration. The oil base is thought to prolong the duration of action.

Drug	Duration	Comparative Potency*
Hydrocortisone	8-12 hrs	1
Prednisone	12-36 hrs	4
Methylprednisone	12-36 hrs	5
Triamcinolone	12-36 hrs	5
Isoflupredone	12-36 hrs	50
Dexamethasone	32-48 hrs	30
Betamethasone	32-48 hrs	30
Flumethasone	>48 hrs	120

* Potency is determined by comparison to a cortisol a value of 1.0.

Corticosteroids and Published Duration of Action.

Drug	Relative Anti-inflammatory Potency	Relative Sodium-retaining Potency	Approximate Duration of Action based on Adrenal Suppression (hr)	Duration of Action (Category)
Cortisol (Hydrocortisone)	1	1	<12	Short acting
Cortisone	0.8	0.8	<12	Short acting
Prednisolone	4	0.8	12-36	Intermediate
Prednisone	4	0.8	12-36	Intermediate
Methylprednisolone	5	0-0.5	12-36	Intermediate (often regarded as drug long acting in joint)
Triamcinolone	3-5	0	24-48	Intermediate
Isoflupredone	17	0	-	Long acting (often regarded as short to intermediate in joint)
Betamethasone	25-30	0	>48	Long acting
Dexamethasone	25-30	0	>48	Long acting
Flumethasone	30	0	>48	Long acting

SYSTEMIC BLOOD AND URINE DRUG LEVELS FOLLOWING INTRA-ARTICULAR CORTICOSTEROID THERAPY

It is important to recognize that numerous factors affect plasma and urinary detection of medications. These factors impose an inherent limitation to the ability to establish universally reliable guidelines regarding drug detection in equine blood and urine samples. Factors such as the rate of urine production, urine pH, intra-horse and inter-horse variability, feeding, diseases, exercise, drug dosage, frequency and route of administration, drug interactions, testing methodology, sample handling and varying formulations of the same medication all impart significant variability to drug detection. The following paragraphs seek to offer information regarding the detection of corticosteroid in blood and urine samples following intra-articular corticosteroid therapy. This information is presented as a guideline only for the selection and timing of intra-articular corticosteroid therapy relative to events that employ drug testing. Despite the numerous variables affecting drug detection, it is generally believed that doubling the dose administered will likely double the peak plasma and urine concentrations and increase the time that the drug will be detectable by one half-life.

The intra-articular administration of triamcinolone acetonide (Vetalog) at a dose of 6 mg to three joints for a total dose of 18 mg was reported to produce detectable serum and synovial fluid concentrations of triamcinolone using radioimmunoassay with a sensitivity of 10 pg/tube. The serum drug levels peaked 4 hr after intra-articular administration, and were undetectable by 3 days. Fifteen days following this total dose per horse, the triamcinolone levels were undetectable in synovial fluid. There was significant variability among horses was observed. Another investigation studied the drug levels using a test dose of 30 mg of intra-articular triamcinolone, HPLC, and a detection limit of 0.1 ng/ml. Peak concentrations of triamcinolone acetonide were recorded at 12 in serum and at 22 in urine. The drug was undetectable in serum by 120 hr (5 days) and in urine by 200 hr (8.3 days) following its intra-articular administration.

Intra-articular administration of 111.2 mg of methylprednisolone acetate (DepoMedrol) was reported to produce detectable levels of hydrolysed active, methylprednisolone less than 5ng/ml in the plasma for only the first 24 hr following the administration and was detectable in synovial fluid for between 5 and 39 days. The parent compound methylprednisolone acetate, was not detected in plasma samples at any time period. The investigation utilized high performance liquid chromatography (HPLC) with a lower level of sensitivity of 2 to3 ng/ml in plasma and 10–20 ng/ml in synovial fluid. This investigation suggested rapid conversion of methylprednisolone acetate to methylprednisolone. Another investigation evaluated the plasma blood levels of methylprednisolone acetate following a 100 mg intra-articular dose of Depo-Medrol and using both enzyme linked immunosorbent assay (ELISA) and HPLC. The reported a lower limit of detection for the ELISA was 2.5 ng/ml and was 10ng/ml for HPLC. While HPLC failed to detect both methylprednisolone acetate and methylprednisolone in the plasma, using ELISA, methylprednisolone acetate or its derivatives were detected until 72 hr after intra-articular administration of methylprednisolone acetate. Synovial fluid samples analyzed using HPLC detected methylprednisolone up to 10 days after administration. Based on these results and on current sampling techniques, it has been suggested that a single 100 mg dose of Depo-Medrol should be administered at least 72 hr prior to any event associated with drug testing in order to avoid a positive blood or urine result. Furthermore, a withholding time would be 8 days following a single 200 mg intra-articular dose of Depo-Medrol has been suggested. Methylprednisolone acetate has been associated with detection times in the urine from 96 hours to 44 days.

There has been little published reports the effects of intra-articular betamethasone on the detection of the drug or its metabolites in equine blood and urine. Reports of detection of betamethasone in general range from 24 hours to over 50 hours depending on route of administration, assay method, dosage. Specific information pertaining to betamethasone and metabolite levels following intra-articular administration in the horse is lacking.

Between 2 and 12 hours after administration of 4 mg of isoflupredone acetate intra-articularly, plasma was found to contain < 10 ng of the drug or any metabolite using an ELISA assay with a sensitivity of 0.1 ng/ml. The parent drug or metabolite equivalent was detected in the urine for 24 hours after intra-articular injection of isoflupredone acetate.

NEGATIVE EFFECTS OF INTRA-ARTICULAR CORTICOSTEROIDS

Despite that corticosteroids are an irreplaceable part of managing joint disease in horses, cavalier use of intra-articular corticosteroid therapy is inadvisable. For reasons already outlined, the public and the equine industry are already likely to be sensitive to the utilization of corticosteroids in the horse. It is therefore imperative that equine veterinarians work sensitively but diligently to educate the public and the industry to the importance of corticosteroid use, while exercising responsible and judicious use of these drugs in their everyday practice.

Joints that have been treated with intra-articular corticosteroids will initially show less pain and swelling than untreated joints. The relief in the clinical signs of joint inflammation will facilitate the desire to return the horse to regular exercise and competition. However, this is not always in the best interest of the horse. It is important that the attending veterinarian be very familiar with the stage and degree of joint inflammation and pathology in order to make appropriate decisions regarding the return of the horse to its regular work. Undiagnosed fractures, cartilage defects, osteochondral fragments and other joint pathologies will greatly add to the damage incurred when the now minimally symptomatic joint is subjected to the return to exercise and the associated mechanical trauma. This results in perpetuation of joint surface damage, reduced joint function and mobility, and ultimately leads to disability of the horse.

Additionally, as our ability to identify soft tissue pathology within and adjacent to joints, the potential for intra-articular steroid to "mask" an underlying soft tissue injury must be considered. Common examples include a temporarily decreased lameness score following injection of a tarsometatarsal joint with steroid when the underlying problem is injury to the proximal suspensory ligament. Similarly, injection of a steroid product into the coffin joint will temporarily reduce lameness scores in horses with injury to the distal deep digital flexor tendon. For this reason, practitioners may choose to wait 21 days before allowing the horse to return to hard work.

As previously discussed, intra-articular corticosteroid usage, particularly that of methylprednisolone, has been reported to be deleterious to the joint through negative effects on chondrocyte metabolism. These effects appear to be prominent at high concentrations where the corticosteroids are capable of inhibiting proteoglycan synthesis and negatively effecting the structural organization of collagen within the joint cartilage. Lower concentrations of corticosteroids are reported to produce these effects reversibly. The corticosteroid levels reported to adversely affect cartilage matrix synthesis appear to exceed those required to inhibit the synthesis of inflammatory and destructive mediators. Although adverse effects occur following repetitive intra-articular injections in exercising horses, the involvement of corticosteroid arthopathy in this is unclear. Nonetheless, it is imperative for the equine practitioner to carefully and completely evaluate all candidates for intra-articular therapy and to utilize judicious and conservative doses and frequency of administration in order to avoid the potential for any damaging effects to the health of the cartilage and overall joint of the recipient horse. In an attempt to minimize the deleterious effects of intra-articular corticosteroids on joint tissues, utilization of the lowest clinically effective dose possible for all intra-articular corticosteroids is recommendable. Unfortunately, the determination of the minimally effective dose for each corticosteroid is presently based on clinical experience and empirical use.

Anytime a joint is entered, there is a risk of infection. This risk increases with administration of corticosteroids or PSGAG. However, infection is rare if good aseptic preparation and technique is utilized in association with minimizing the number of attempts to enter a joint. With good preparation technique, clipping of the hair over the site of entry is generally regarded as unnecessary unless the area has long hair and/or is abnormally dirty. Many clients will request the veterinarian to NOT clip to avoid the obvious cosmetic implications. In reality, veterinarians are routinely expected to inject joints in sub-optimal environment where factors such as: dirty floor, wind and confined work place etc make the true asepsis impossible to achieve. As veterinarians, we are forced to deal with these scenarios as they arise. Because of this, many practitioners add an antimicrobial to their intra-articular medication to minimize the likelihood of post injection sepsis. Other equine practitioners rarely combine antimicrobials with the corticosteroid unless they perceive an increased risk of infection in association with a particular clinical situation. Furthermore, the administration of amikacin into a joint may be argued to be a risk factor for the development of post-injection aseptic synovitis (joint flare). There has been speculation that joints with severe osteoarthritis may be more prone to post-injection sepsis. Combining antimicrobials with intra-articular medication may be warranted when treating such joints. At this time, amikacin is the antimicrobial of choice to be added to the IA medication. Although gentamicin was used previously, it has become popular to administer in this manner. Although less expensive than amikacin, gentamicin has a narrower spectrum of activity as well as possibly creating a higher incidence of "joint flare".

Laminitis is an important consideration anytime a corticosteroid is administered by any route. The incidence of laminitis in association with intra-articular corticosteroid administration is likely to be less than parenteral administration. Nonetheless, there is very strong belief that triamcinolone is capable of inducing laminitis in horses after intra-articular administration if excessive doses are utilized. For this reason, some equine practitioners avoid the use of triamcinolone, some do not exceed certain pre-determined doses, some will not use the drug in more than one joint, some will not use it more than once on an individual horse on an individual day, and some will not administer the drug in excess of a certain dose or in combination with any other corticosteroid administration.The incidence of laminitis secondary to administrationof triamcinolone at doses two to four times greater than that used by most practitioners resulted in a low occurrence of laminitis. Some practitioners report rarely experiencing laminitis when a utilizing a cautious standard dose and frequency for horses that do not have other metabolic problems or a history of laminitis. Regardless, it is advisable to approach any corticosteroid administration, intra-articular and otherwise, with similar caution. Although laminitis is a potentially devastating risk factor to be considered when using triamcinolone in middle age and older horses, triamcinolone remains one of the most effective and potentially beneficial intra-articular medications available to the practitioner.

INTRA-ARTICULAR SILICONE

The use of intra-articular silicone has been reported in Standardbred racehorses in conjunction with corticosteroids in order to treat unresponsive joint disease. Liquid silicone fluid is reported to be chemically inert, hydrophobic, and to exhibit low volatility, resistance to decomposition by heat, low surface tension and a wide range of viscosity. These characteristics were regarded as potentially beneficial for its use as an intra-articular therapy for horses. However, investigations into the effects of medical grade silicone into normal carpal joints found that silicone caused an acute synovitis when injected intra-articularly. It was subsequently phagocytized by macrophages and incorporated in the subsynovium with minimal chronic synovial inflammatory response, while clinical signs of joint disease (effusion, lameness) persisted. In these investigations, single intra-articular administration of two milliliters of medical grade liquid silicone did not result in appreciable articular cartilage damage six weeks after administration. Furthermore, the efficacy of liquid silicone as an exogenous lubricant is questionable. The lubrication of articular cartilage (at low loads) and soft tissues is normally accomplished by the binding of lubricin and hyaluronic acid. These molecules prevent direct contact of opposing surfaces and thereby, decrease the coefficient of friction between two opposing surfaces. The phagocytosis of liquid silicone by intrasynovial macrophages and its removal from synovial fluid preclude its ability to function as a lubricant. Silicone appears to induce an acute synovitis when injected into an equine joint and clinical signs of joint disease (joint circumference, effusion, lameness) persist after injection. Therefore, despite that liquid silicone did not appear to result in appreciable articular cartilage, at this time, the degree of acute synovitis and apparent inability to function as a lubricant precludes a recommendation to utilize this compound for intra-articular therapy of joint disease in the horse.

TILDURONATE (TILDREN)

In some countries, Tiludronate is approved for intravenous use in horses. Tildren has been shown to be a potent bone pain inhibitor by means of osteoclast inhibition. The beneficial effect following intravenous administration can be anticipated to last at least 6 months. Some practitioners use tiludronate intra-articularly with apparently no negative side effects. Dosage of intra-articular Tildren has not been established, although practitioners report using 1 of the 10 ml vials into the affected joint following normal joint preparation. Its efficacy as an intra-articular medication has not yet been evaluated.

PLATELET-RICH PLASMA (PRP)

Platelet-rich plasma has been used in human medicine primarily for reconstructive surgery and wound care. Platelets contain numerous growth factors as inflammatory mediators. Intra-articular PRP has been anecdotally reported to have been used successfully in horses. Its comparative value is unknown at this time. PRP is most likely to be of value as an IA therapy in treatment of an acute injury to the joint.

JOINT INJECTION OF THE AXIAL SEKELETON

Recent advances in imaging techniques have helped veterinarians identify sources of pain or arthritis within joints of the axial skeleton. Most commonly the intervertebral dorsal articular facet (DAF) joints, can cause significant performance impairment and, to a lesser extent, lameness. Ultrasound guided injection of these joints is performed routinely.

Unique to these joints is the proximity to the spinal canal and its contents. In theory, products injected into the facet joint of the axial skeleton may "leak" into the CSF. For this reason, relatively small volumes are recommended, and the inclusion of sarapin is to be conducted with caution. Additionally, there are anecdotal reports of technique failure where the spinal needle punctures the spinal cord during DAF injection (under ultrasound guidance). Similarly, strict attention to aseptic technique is necessary.

INTRA-ARTICULAR INJECTION TECHNIQUE

Although joints of the distal limb are routinely injected, occasionally a specific joint may be difficult to enter. This may be due to regional scar tissue, patient non compliance, previous periarticular injections or other reasons. The practitioner is encouraged to visualize synovial fluid when injecting a joint. Occasionally, despite being in the joint, digital pressure to the surrounding region is needed to fill the needle hub with synovial fluid. In other instances, the sound of air rushing thru the injection needle once the joint is entered will suggest proper needle placement. Occasionally, neither of the above mentioned indicators is present, and the practitioner must rely on the characteristic "feel" of non resistance as the product is injected. Finally, the use of digital radiology and/or ultrasonography may be beneficial in identifying landmarks for needle placement.

The equine practitioner is expected to make significant efforts to achieve aseptic preparation of the injection site. This includes surgical scrub of the area injection site with an antimicrobial soap and alcohol. Clipping of the injection site is optimal, but not routinely done in equine practice unless the area is especially dirty or the hair is exceptionally long. Use of non-reusable latex gloves is also standard practice. When synovial fluid is visualized during the injection, the veterinarian may comment on the volume, color and/or viscosity or "string" of the fluid. Excessive synovial pressure appears to correlate with joint pain and inflammation. The appearance of decreased synovial viscosity may be a normal finding in the low hock joints and the coffin joint.

INTRA-ARTICULAR INJECTION AFTERCARE

A light bandage is often placed over the injection site. Application of an antimicrobial ointment or spray onto the injection site following injection is also considered to be routine, particularly following injection of the foot region. Oral phenylbutazone (or another NSAID) may be prescribed for a few days in order to reduce the incidence of joint flare. Alternatively, some veterinarians prefer to utilize topical diclofenac sodium (Surpass) over the joint to control post-injection inflammation. Most horses receive stall rest and hand walking for varying amounts of time following intra-articular therapy. Some clinicians and researchers advocate 10–14 days of stall and run confinement followed by a gradual return to full work during the subsequent week, as a post-intra-articular corticosteroid exercise protocol. A minimum rest period is probably important, but extended rest is often impractical for the client expectations and competition schedule. Some situations demand abbreviated rest of a few days (1 to 3 days) before beginning a gradual return to regular work. Most horses are not worked for at least 1 week following injection, although an extended rest is not recommended unless the problem in the joint warrants a period of inactivity. Specifically, if the practitioner is considering an injury to a soft tissue structure near the joint in question, it is advisable to avoid hard work for 21 days following the injection when possible. Intra-articular therapies are often combined with systemic therapies such as intravenous hyaluronan, intramuscular polysulfated glycosaminoglycans, nutraceutical compounds and/or other ancillary therapies.

DETERMINING IF INTRA-ARTICULAR INJECTION IS INDICATED

In many parts of the world, the sport horse show industry is extremely competitive. Livelihoods depend in part on the success of the trainer/rider in the show arena. In the past, sporthorse veterinarians were unlikely to treat a joint in a leg without confirming the diagnosis via a nerve block and some form of imaging. Today, however, many trainers have had extensive firsthand experience with not only training, but also the benefits of intra-articular treatment of their horses. Many successful trainers seek a “competitive edge” which may involve some form of intra-articular therapy. In today’s competition circuits, it is not uncommon for a trainer/rider to request a joint injection without any form of veterinary examination. Although trainers may have extensive experience with intra-articular therapies, they may not be aware of any negative effects or risks associated with such therapies. This scenario presents ethical and a potential liability issue to the sporthorse veterinarian. The trainer may think the horse needs a “maintainence” injection. The veterinarian must decide whether to rely on the trainers expertise in identifying when and where the horse is sore, or to require some form of examination leading to a veterinary opinion. Trainers may become frustrated if, after a thorough examination, the veterinarian cannot definitively identify a specific joint problem or injury. The veterinarian may become frustrated if he/she feels pressure to treat a joint unnecessarily, the trainer demands treatment of what the veterinarian considers to be the wrong joint, the veterinarian feels a critical soft tissue injury is the real problem, or if a complication to the injection occurs and the owner (not the trainer) cannot understand why the joint was treated without prior examination.

At this time, agreeing to inject a horses joint at the request of a trainer or owner is done on a routine basis by many sporthorse veterinarians, provided that there is a strong relationship between the sporthorse trainer/owner and the veterinarian. The relationship and the shared experiences with joint injections presumes that the trainer is knowledgeable about the relevant diagnostic and therapeutic options, and has been made aware of the basic risks associated with intraarticular procedures. The veterinarian agree to forego an examination prior to treatment in an effort to save the client the expense of the examination and/or the cost of additional diagnostic tools. It is not within the scope of this chapter to review the ethical or legal ramifications of this scenario. It is the authors intentions to identify this dilemma which the sporthorse veterinarian may routinely face, and that many practitioners will inject horses joints at the request of a trainer/owner without actually examining the horse. Each veterinarian must decide on an individual basis what an appropriate and professional response is to this request.

The utilization of intra-articular injection has increased with the changes in expectations of our clients and the progression of articular management strategies. It is now common to utilize intra-articular injection techniques in the diagnosis of lameness, management of joint sepsis, and in the management and control of the progression of joint disease including degenerative joint disease. In subclinical lameness issues, (not lame enough to "block"), identifying an improvement following injection of a specific joint may support the diagnosis of joint pain. However, injuries to soft tissue structures will frequently improve following injection of an adjacent joint.

To a large extent, focus has moved from treating existing lameness to detecting joint problems early in the developmental process. Many trainers and owners have had firsthand experiences where their horses results and longevity improved dramatically following IA therapy. Similarly some horses may experience secondary tendonitis/desmitis (eg. the horse injures a front SDF tendon or injures a suspensory ligament presumably because the opposite front leg or diagonal hindlimb has a low grade lameness). As the horse protects the low grade primary problem, the horse overloads and injures the previously unaffected leg. Some trainers may not perceive a significant potential for negative sequelae to IA therapy, and therefore have a cavalier approach to IA therapy. Similarly, some riders may seek veterinary therapies to remedy non-veterinary problems (ineffective training and conditioning methods etc). For this reason, it is advisable to assess the potential risks of IA therapy vs. the real indications for intra-articular injection. As a rule, it is advisable for the clinician to have "a specific reason" to inject a horse's joint. Reasons may include: lameness, positive response to flexion tests, imaging findings, physical exam findings, history or request of a trainer/ professional. Hopefully, when deciding to inject a joint, the "best interest of the horse" is the primary objective of all parties involved.

Performance horse veterinarians are commonly faced with horses affected with synovitis and capsulitis and that may not exhibit clinical signs other than reduced level of performance. Common muscle and other soft-tissue soreness in horses can significantly add to the ambiguity that relates to the detection of an early lameness problem that may require or benefit from some intervention. At this time, equine veterinarians must rely on their experience, hands and eyes in order to evaluate and diagnose joint and soft tissue problems of the equine locomotor apparatus. An astute practitioner may add to his/her evaluation by watching the horse exercise and/or during competition. History, physical examination, palpation and manipulation and flexion findings are added to develop a case for the need to intervene with intra-articular injection techniques. Using these examination approaches, performance horse veterinarians are detecting joints with synovitis and capsulitis that can be associated with inadequate performance.

Horses that are presented with obvious lameness and synovial effusion are more likely to exhibit more advanced joint disease. However, facilitating the recognition and presentation of a horse in the early stages of a joint problem may prove to be a problem. Therefore, performance horse veterinarians should strive to become more regularly involved in coordinated management of the maintenance of performance, routine lameness evaluation and management of overall joint health. Such increased interaction facilitates coordination with the client and caregivers in early detection and intervention when a joint problem is still in the early stages. The rapidly expanding armamentarium of diagnostic and therapeutic techniques and technology is also enabling the performance horse veterinarian to more completely evaluate and manage horses in the early stages of soft tissue and joint problems that may limit performance as well as horses with chronic and significant lameness problems. These technologies and techniques are well recognized by equine practitioners.

The decision of when to use intra-articular corticosteroids to manage horses with joint disease must be made on a case by case basis. Intra-articular medication is generally preferred over systemic treatment because it appears to be more effective at reducing the clinical signs of joint disease. Therefore, utilizing intra-articular corticosteroids is no longer be regarded as a last resort to manage horses with joint problems. In fact, the disease modifying characteristics of corticosteroids are now recognized as important tools in the control and management of equine joint inflammation and the progression of joint disease. Once they are detected, synovitis and capsulitis are often treated with intra-articular hyaluronic acid alone or more often in combination with a corticosteroid. The combination of intra-articular corticosteroids with hyaluronan is now used routinely to manage horses with joint disease. The primary exceptions probably include the management of osteoarthritis of the distal tarsal joints where the benefit of using HA is unclear. As a general guideline in the selection of an appropriate corticosteroid, many performance horse veterinarians tend to utilize triamcinolone acetate or betamethasone acetate/phosphate in high-motion joints (all joints other than the distal tarsal joints) specifically for the combination of their disease modifying and anti-inflammatory effects, and methylprednisolone acetate in low-motion joints such as the distal tarsal joints.

JOINT BIOMARKERS

Biomarkers are believed to be molecular messengers involved in various homeostatic and disease processes. Their expression may be quantified and utilized to identify disruption in homeostasis and progression of disease. Recognized joint "biomarkers" include the precursors of two major components of cartilage; collagen and aggrecan. When aggrecan is being synthesized, a portion of a precursor molecule is released; an increase in the concentration of that portion indicates that aggrecan synthesis is increasing. Similarly, a precursor of collagen can be detected when collagen is being synthesized. These molecular biomarkers can help distinguish between synthesis and degradation of the cartilage matrix markers. Concentrations of these biomarkers increase further in the presence of joint disease. These markers might thereby be used to differentiate disease processes and to monitor the progression of those processes. Despite this potential application, the interpretation of the levels of biomarkers is complicated by the fact that that they change with age and level of exercise Thus, biomarker levels are different in young and old horses, and basal levels are higher in horses undergoing athletic activities.

In clinical trials in which biomarkers were compared in joint fluid and serum samples from horses undergoing arthroscopy and horses in the general population, samples of joint fluid or serum were effectively used to differentiate the two populations of horses with approximately 79% certainty. Furthermore, the researchers were also able to stage the disease by the concentration of the biomarker and to identify different patterns or averages for each of the disease processes. The proposed utility of these findings is the potential to define a predictive index that could help identify horses with specific problems. Clinical situations are far more complex than experimentally induced joint disease, but there is hope to make further the understanding of this technology and perhaps to make it commercially to monitor treatment and disease progression.

Complications of Equine Joint Injection

Infection

Any intra-articular procedure is associated with the potential to introduce bacteria into the joint. However, with proper preparation and sterile technique, the risk of infection is minimized. Even with the best of limb preparation and sterile technique, there remains some risk of infection with intra-articular injection. The risk of infection increases with the administration of intra-articular corticosteroids and polysulfated glycosaminoglycans, and with repeated attempts to enter the target joint.

The symptoms of joint infection and joint "flare" are similar; heat, swelling and tenderness around the joint, reluctance to use the affected limb normally. Therefore, differentiating between sepsis and flare based on clinical signs is not always clear. Little published information exists to help specifically differentiate between clinical signs of joint sepsis and joint flare. Ultimately, analysis of synovial fluid from the affected joint may be the most definitive answer. Characteristically, the clinical signs of a septic joint will rapidly worsen and the horse displays severe lameness within 24 hours of onset of clinical signs. Even in the face of aggressive antibiotic therapy, a joint infection may cause extensive destruction of the articular cartilage and may result in significant lameness or permanent loss of use. If a joint is becomes infected, there is often some time delay to the onset of clinical signs (5-15 days because the corticosteroid has suppressed the inflammatory process during the early phases of infection), and the onset of symptoms can be rapid and severe. In contrast, symptoms of joint "flare" typically occur within 3 days of joint injection and tend to respond to NSAIDS and physical therapies. Elevated body temperatures can be seen in both scenarios.

If joint sepsis is suspected, aggressive diagnostics and interventions are warranted. This includes blood work, synoviocentesis with cytological evaluation and joint fluid culture, aggressive systemic antimicrobial therapy, joint lavage, regional limb perfusion, intra-articular antimicrobial administration and effective pain management. Assessment of synovial fluid may reveal elevated WBC and protein values, "degenerative" neutrophils, and presence of bacteria. For more specific laboratory values, consult an equine surgery reference. The clinician must also be careful to distinguish celulitis-like problems from joint sepsis. Synoviocentesis through inflammed tissue may result in introduction of septic material into the joint environment.

Masking Pain/ Facilitating Continued Exercise

Injecting corticosteroids into a damaged joint can help reduce inflammation and relieve pain, but they may increase the risk for re-injury or worsening of the joint pathology when the horse returns to work. Appropriate evaluation of the affected joint, judicious use of corticosteroids and good post-injection management is necessary in order to help prevent this unwanted outcome. (see above references to IA cortisone therapy "masking" adjacent soft tissue injuries)

Broken Needles

In very rare instances of intra-articular injection, a needle may break and part of the needle remain in the horse. The likelihood of such an occurrence has decreased significantly with the advent of more flexible alloy needles in comparison to the much more brittle stainless steel needles of the past. Larger gauge needles are less likely to break, however they are more painful to the horse during injection. Additionally, proper sedation and manual restraint can help reduce the likelihood of breaking a needle during injection. If a needle breaks in a joint, it is important to assess the situation radiographically. If the needle is in contact with articular cartilage, it will likely require surgical removal. Occasionally, a needle fragment resides in surrounding connective tissue which may not require removal. Such decisions are made on an individual basis.

Reactive Synovitis (Joint Flare)

This complication is generally the most common complication following intra-articular injection. "Flare" is a chemically induced synovitis resulting from introduction of any foreign substance into a joint. "joint flare" result from a inflammatory response to the medication, to the "carrying vehicles", to buffering or to preservative products within a given IA formulation. Theoretically, "joint flare" may also occur if foreign material such as dirt, hair or a counterirritant is introduced into the joint. It is widely considered that by administering NSAIDS and halting exercise following IA injection, the likelihood of "flare" is decreased. Long term effects of a single "flare' episode are generally considered not significant. However, the clinician should be careful not to repeat the use of the same product in the joint of concern if possible. Of primary concern is the diagnosis and differentiation of a reactive synovitis from joint sepsis. The occurrence of either of these complications mandates immediate attention and diagnostics to clearly outline the exact etiology of the complication. The following section discusses the appropriate considerations and approaches required to make this determination.

Cartilage Damage

As previously discussed, there is a significant body of evidence to suggest that cavalier use of intra-articular corticosteroids is associated with cartilage damage. Although complete avoidance of intra-articular corticosteroid use is also not supportive of overall joint health, judicious utilization of these powerful anti-inflammatory drugs can be tremendously valuable. The potential for cartilage damage may vary with the frequency of administration, the drug used and the doses administered. As such, the lowest effective dose of corticosteroid is advised. Furthermore, based on the current understanding of the corticosteroids used for intra-articular injection, it is probably worthwhile to utilize triamcinolone or betamethasone for high motion joints due to their purported and relative "cartilage sparing" effects.

Laminitis

While corticosteroids (intra-articular and/or systemic) are important for controlling and treating joint disease in the horse, there is significant anecdotal evidence to indicate that steroids, especially triamcinolone, may contribute to the onset of laminitis. Minimizing the doses utilized, the number of corticosteroid drugs used at the same time and establishing an upper limit dosage for triamcinolone, administered alone or with other corticosteroid administration, is advisable and may help to minimize liability and to maximize the perception of attention given to this concern.

Diagnosis and Differentiation of Joint Flare (Reactive Synovitis) from Joint Sepsis

The incidence of post-injection flare has been reported to be about 2%, but probably varies widely depending on which product are administered, aftercare, injection technique, and which joints are predominantly injected at a given practice. Post-injection flare is difficult to distinguish clinically from intra-articular sepsis. While any entry into a joint will induce some degree of synovitis, an injected medication and/or its vehicle my further induce a chemical synovitis. Contamination of intra-articular medications with bacteria and/or endotoxin can cause reactive synovitis or joint contamination and sepsis. Such contamination may be more commonly encountered if multiple intra-articular doses are harvested from the same medication vial, and if the vial is repeatedly used for more than one horse, and/or is used on more than one occasion. Bacteria and/or debris can also be carried into the joint during IA injection whether the joint has been aseptically prepared or not. Obviously, aseptic technique dramatically reduces the amount of contaminants introduced into the joint. Standard aseptic technique may or may not include local clipping the area to be injected. Appropriate aspetic technique should must includeuse of an antimicrobial scrub soap (typically betadine or chlorhexadine), followed by an alcohol rinse and removal of soap residues just prior to injection. Typically, 3 cycles of soap and alcohol are used. Optimally, the scrub soap will have 10 minutes of exposure time to kill the microbes on the skin. In addition to this technique, many veterinarians refuse to utilize previously opened bottles of intra-articular medication and demand to open the bottle for the first time immediately prior to the any intra-articular injection. The routine utilization of sterile gloves for any intra-articular injection is strongly recommended.

It has been shown that following intra-articular injection of methylprednisolone acetate, inflammatory cells are found to surround crystals of the vehicle that are imbedded within the synovium. A joint flare can occur if the body reacts to the injected product as a foreign substance or if the product acts as an irritant. In such cases, the flare often subsides following anti-inflammatory therapy with or without joint lavage to facilitate crystal removal. With a joint flare long-term problems are uncommon. However, this reactive synovitis may lead to enough increase in circulation of the joint such that the medication administered is effectively removed, leading to ineffective treatment. Eosinophilic synovitis has been reported, but appears to be rare. It has been postulated to be associated with an allergic reaction to an injected product or to be idiopathic. Anecdotally, joint flare is believed to be most common with methylprednisolone acetate. Furthermore, the distal interphalangeal joint and the tarsocrural joint have been reported to be at increased risk for developing reactive synovitis following injcction with polysulfated glysosaminoglycans. The tarsocrural joint is the joint may be more susceptible to joint flare following injection.

It is important to distinguish joint flare from septic arthritis. The initial clinical presentation of a "flare" and a "sepsis" can be indistinguishable. With joint flare, horses may show signs of mild to severe lameness from within hours to a few days after the injection. The distinguishing features suggesting reactive synovitis include an early onset after injection, synovial nucleated cell counts of less than 30,000/μl, and partial resolution within 1 to 3 days. The septic synovial fluid typically has a predominant presence of neutrophils (90%) and those cells frequently appear "unhealthy" on cytologic evaluation. Synovial fluid following joint flare typically has fewer neutrophils than in septic fluid, (70%) with an increase in monocytes (30%). An inflammatory process in a structure near a joint may cause transient increase in synovial fluid WBC numbers. Septic synovial fluid will usually contain bacteria on cytological examination. The most definitive tool for differentiation is synovial fluid analysis. Systemic antimicrobial therapy can be of great value in treatment of early septic arthritis. It is possible that some horses which have been considered to be "flare" cases and treated with antimicrobials, were actually low level septic and respond favorably to the antimicrobial therapy.

The clinician must weigh the risks of synoviocentesis against the necessity for the diagnosis. Joint sepsis may occur 1/10 as frequently as joint flare. For this reason, whether the joint is infected or is exhibiting a "flare", antibiotics and NSAID therapy is instituted immediately after examination. If immediate synoviocentesis is performed, it is performed prior to therapy. If the horse responds significantly to conservative therapy within 24 hours of treatment, it is more likely to be a joint flare. If the reaction occurs 10 or more days following IA cortisone injection, there is a much higher likelihood of joint sepsis.

Introduction of IA corticosteroid may prolong the time to manifestation of clinical symptoms associated with joint sepsis. In these instances, the horse's ability to mount a normal immune defense is compromised. Clinical symptoms become apparent when bacterial counts are high, and the disease process has become well established within the joint. Therefore, sepsis following IA injection with steroid will appear later (7-14) days following the injection. The horse will usually deteriorate rapidly (over 24 hours) following the initial symptoms to display profound discomfort and eventually non-weight bearing lameness. Following an injury where a joint capsule has been lacerated and surgically closed,, it can take up to 14 days following surgical closure before signs of joint sepsis are recognized. Prompt management with intra-articular lavage, systemic and local antimicrobial drug administration and anti-inflammatory therapy is recommended for a septic joint. Culture and sensitivity testing should be performed on the joint fluid. This condition is similarly managed.

Broken needles, plant or seed awns, thorns and cactus spines, debris from nearby wounds may also lead to reactive synovitis or sepsis. These etiologies should be considered in the evaluation of reactive synovitis following intra-articular injection.

Conclusion

Intra-articular injections have become an integral part of performance horse practice. Although the entry of a joint with a needle imparts some risk, appropriate preparation and injection techniques and medication use minimize the occurrence of post-injection reactions such as non-septic, reactive synovitis (joint flare) and joint sepsis. With the increased utilization of intra-articular injection, medications for intra-articular administration have been more completely investigated and new medications and therapies have been introduced for intra-articular use. Of particular prominence in the advancement of intra-articular therapy has been the increased focus on Disease Modifying Osteoarthritis Drugs (DMOADs). It is particularly interesting to recognize that despite their history of reported significant negative characteristics, intra-articular corticosteroids are now well recognized as an important and powerful class of drugs that benefit joints that are inflamed when they are used judiciously. Corticosteroids are therefore now considered to exhibit DMOAD properties and represent potent and economical way of helping to control and manage synovitis and osteoarthritis in the horse.

References

[1] Autefage A, Alvinerie M, Toutain PL. *Synovial fluid and plasma kinetics of methylprednisolone and methylprednisolone acetate in horses following intra-articular administration of methylprednisolone acetate*. Equine Vet J, 1986 May;18(3):193-8.

[2] Caron JP. *Intra-articular injections for joint disease in horses*. Vet Clin North Am Equine Pract, 2005 Dec;21(3):559-73, v.

[3] Caron JP. *Large Animal Veterinary Rounds*: Therapy for Equine Joint Disease. 2006. Available from: www.canadianveterinarians.net/larounds

[4] Caron JP, Genovese RL. *Principles and practices of joint disease.* In: Ross MW, Dyson SJ, editors. Diagnosis and management of lameness in the horse. Philadelphia, Pa.: London; 2003.

[5] Carter J, Carter GK, Easter JL, Frisbie D, McClure S, Mitchell RD. *Managing equine joint inflammation: A roundtable discussion on diagnostic and treatment options*. Suppl Compend Cont Ed Pract Vet; Equine Edition 2(3)A; 2007; 1-16.

[6] Dowling PM. *Myths and truths about controlling pain and inflammation in horses:* Proceedings of the Alberta horse breeders and owners conference; 1997.

[7] Frisbie DD. *New research and regulatory issue associated with corticosteroids.* AAEP Proceedings 46; 2000; 234-242.

[8] Frisbie DD, Ghivizzani SC, Robbins PD, Evans CH, McIlwraith CW. *Treatment of experimental equine osteoarthritis by in vivo delivery of the equine interleukin-1 receptor antagonist gene*. Gene Ther, 2002 Jan;9(1):12-20.

[9] Frisbie DD, Ray CS, Ionescu M, Poole AR, Chapman PL, McIlwraith CW. *Measurement of synovial fluid and serum concentrations of the 846 epitope of chondroitin sulfate and of carboxy propeptides of type II procollagen for diagnosis of osteochondral fragmentation in horses.* Am J Vet Res, 1999 Mar;60(3):306-9.

[10] Gerken DF, Sams RA. *Factors affecting drug withholding time estimates in horses.* Vet Clin North Am Equine Pract, 1993 Dec;9(3):461-79.

[11] Koupai-Abyazani MR, Yu N, Esaw B, Laviolette B. *Determination of triamcinolone acetonide in equine serum and urine by liquid chromatography-atmospheric pressure ionization mass spectrometry.* J Anal Toxicol, 1995 May-Jun;19(3):182-6.

[12] Lillich JD, Bertone AL, Schmall LM, Ruggles AJ, Sams RA. *Plasma, urine, and synovial fluid disposition of methylprednisolone acetate and isoflupredone acetate after intra-articular administration in horses.* Am J Vet Res, 1996 Feb;57(2):187-92.

[13] Rumbaugh ML. *The effects of intra-articular silicone polymer on synovial fluid, synovial tissue and articular cartilage in the equine middle carpal joint.* Thesis; Graduate Faculty of the Louisiana State University and Agricultural and Mechanical College in partial fulfillment of the requirements for the degree of Master of Science: 2003.

[14] Unknown. *Corticosteroid - glucocorticoid effects (Veterinary—Systemic);* The United States Pharmacopeial Convention: 2004; 1-67.

In: Rehabilitating the Athletic Horse
Editors: H. W. Jann et al., pp. 117-158
ISBN: 978-1-678-1-60876-672-7

Chapter 7

EXTRA-ARTICULAR THERAPIES USED IN THE MANAGEMENT OF LAMENESS

***Bradford G. Bentz*[1] *and Mark S. Revenaugh*[2]**
[1]VMD, MS, DACVIM, ACVP (Equine), Hagyard Equine Medical Institute in Lexington, Kentucky, USA
[2]DVM. Northwest Equine Performance LLC, Mulino, OR, USA

ABSTRACT

In addition to intra-articular therapies covered in a previous chapter, there are also a large number of other procedures that do not involve intra-articular injection. The goals of these therapies vary with the condition(s) being addressed, and as with intra-articular injection, the ability to meet these goals is heavily dependent on the completeness of the diagnostic approach and the accuracy of the diagnosis.

INTRODUCTION

Many of the therapies discussed in this chapter are well recognized and validated treatments. However, in performance horse practice there has evolved a number of other therapeutic approaches that are supported primarily by experience of repeatable clinical efficacy and/or owner/trainer/rider reported clinical benefit. These therapies have increased in number in the last several years with increasing client expectations, in response to changing restrictions imposed by drug testing and with increased experience and willingness of the sport horse veterinarian to embrace less well recognized treatment approaches for a variety of performance horse problems.

Disease Modifying Osteoarthritis Drugs and Symptom Modifying Osteoarthritis Drugs

As described in human medicine, there are two major drug categories that are most commonly utilized in thetreatment and control of to osteoarthritis.. These are the symptom-modifying osteoarthritis drugs (SMOADs) and the disease-modifying osteoarthritis drugs (DMOADs). In general, SMOADs alleviate pain that produce improvement in clinical signs , such as reduction in lameness and response to flexion. DMOADs however actually affect the degenerative process and thereby slow the progression of joint deterioration. Not all DMOADs exhibit symptom-modifying effects. Therefore, the most beneficial treatment requires the use of a drug or drug combination that exhibits the characteristics of both drug categories. Currently a common approach is intra-articular steroid administration, specifically triamcinolone, which has both disease- and symptom-modifying effects. However, high doses or long-term use of intra-articular triamcinolone (or other intra-articular medications) may be associated with adverse events. Therefore non-articular therapeutic options to symptom-modifying and disease-modifying drug properties drugs are being actively investigated and marketed. Drugs such as intravenous hyaluronic acid and intramuscular polysufated glycosaminoglycan are being developed to offer symptom and disease-modifying effects. Treatment modalities, such as shock-wave therapy, Interleukin 1 Receptor Antagonist Protein (IRAP) and topical diclofenac, among others, have been associated with some decrease in thc progression of joint conditions and clinical improvement. Further research isplanned or underway in order to more specifically, evaluate various medications and interventions for disease-modifying effects. .

Non-Steroidal Anti-Inflammatory Drugs (NSAIDS)

Phenylbutazone (PBZ), flunixin meglumine, meclofenamate and ketoprofen are the most commonly administered NSAIDs for the elimination and control of musculoskeletal pain and inflammation. Although it is easy to engage in cavalier administer of these medications for most musculoskeletal conditions, it is important to recognize that they are associated with significant and potentially severe side-effects including gastrointestinal ulceration and reductions in kidney perfusion. Because of these potential side-effects, systemic NSAID administration is not recommended at high doses or for prolonged periods of time. It is also appropriate to strongly consider some preventive therapy for gastrointestinal ulceration anytime an NSAID is administered to a horse. In situations that may require prolonged or high doses of NSAIDs in order to help control pain or lameness, it is important to further consider the use of other less toxic and perhaps more intensively analgesic therapies. It is also important to evaluate the patient for a condition that may respond more effectively to direct treatment of the underlying problem (such as intra-articular therapies). However, it is important to recognize and to employ the utility of NSAIDs for musculoskeletal pain that may not require intra-articular therapy. The NSAIDs used in horses do not exhibit identical pharmacologic properties and toxicological profiles.

The NSAIDs commonly used in horses include; aspirin, phenylbutazone, dipyrone, flunixin meglumine, meclofenamic acid, firocoxib and ketoprofen. As a group, NSAIDs are weak acids and exhibit high protein binding in blood. Although they are well absorbed from the stomach, the high protein binding in the blood means that most of the drug remains in the blood. Only low levels of NSAIDs are found in normal tissues and joint fluid and these levels are derived from the much smaller fraction of free NSAID in the blood. In damaged tissues and joints however, because of increased blood flow and fluid leakage from the vessels due to inflammation, NSAID levels increase to therapeutic levels. Because NSAIDs are highly bound to blood proteins, caution must be used when other highly protein bound drugs are administered. Competition for protein binding sites can result in dramatic increases in free drug available for pharmacological action of NSAIDs, leading to toxicity. NSAIDs should be administered cautiously to dehydrated horses. Blood concentrations will be greater than normal in the dehydrated horse and are more likely to cause toxicity. Furthermore, renal perfusion is already impaired by hypovolemia and the effects of high doses of NSAIDs will further significantly reduce renal perfusion.

The practice of concurrent administration of two different NSAIDs has received significant attention (aka “stacking”). The premise behind this approach is the presumption of improved anti-inflammatory effect and/or pain relief in comparison to administration of either medication alone. This presumption has been supported in a few studies that have evaluated the co-administration of phenylbutazone and fluinixin meglumine and phynylbutazone and ketoprofen. The concerns for the utilization of this practice include the intensity of analgesia provided that could lead to injury to a horse that otherwise may not have been able to compete or exercise to at a level that would produce an injury and the well documented increase in toxicity seen with coadministration of 2 NSAIDs. Although this practice is currently permitted by the USEF (except for the concurrent use of phenlybutazone and flunixin meglumine), these concerns are being currently undergoing re-evaluation through further research and debate by veterinarians and regulating bodies.

Since all NSAIDs act by the same mechanism of cyclooxygenase inhibition, higher dose of a single NSAID should produce the same response. The NSAIDs block the cyclooxygenase enzyme, interrupting formation of thromboxane, prostacyclin and the prostaglandins from arachidonic acid. This results in antipyretic action (reduces fever), mild pain relief, anti-inflammatory effects and inhibition of platelet clumping. NSAIDs have recently been reported to act on pain receptors in the central nervous system to block pain in the same way as drugs like morphine. NSAIDs may alter immune system responses and suppress inflammatory mediators other than the cyclooxygenase products.

Aspirin

Aspirin has the weakest anti-inflammatory and analgesic (pain relieving) activity of the NSAIDs in horses, so it is rarely used in horses for inflammatory conditions. While the action of most of the other NSAIDs on platelet cyclooxygenase is reversible, aspirin irreversibly binds to cyclooxygenase in platelets and has the greatest anti-clotting activity of the NSAIDs. Its anti-clotting action may be useful in treating conditions in the horse that involve damage to blood vessels and clot formation such as; laminitis, thromboembolic colic and other vascular accidents, recurrent uveitis, and endotoxemia. Aspirin is partially converted in the blood and by the liver to salicylic acid, and this is rapidly excreted by the kidneys into the urine. Salicylic acid is a natural component of horse urine, but the normal concentration is quite low. Drug testing for aspirin requires accounting for this natural production.

Phenylbutazone

Phenylbutazone (PBZ) has analgesic, anti-inflammatory, and antipyretic activity from inhibition of cyclooxygenase. The injectable formulation must be administered by careful intravenous administration only because this formulation causes severe tissue damage if given intramuscularly or subcutaneously. Following oral administration, PBZ is well absorbed, but the time it takes to reach peak blood levels is delayed by feeding. In the blood, greater than 99% of the PBZ is carried bound to blood proteins. Phenylbutazone is converted by the liver to oxyphenbutazone, a metabolite with the same action as PBZ, but this form is removed slower from the body than PBZ. The capacity of the liver to process PBZ becomes overwhelmed at relatively low drug doses. Therefore, increasing doses of PBZ can easily result in toxicity. In the horse, the therapeutic effect of PBZ lasts for more than 24 hours, due to the slow excretion of the oxyphenbutazone metabolite. PBZ and oxyphenbutazone will cross the placenta and are excreted in mare's milk.

The absorption of phenylbutazone from the gastrointestinal tract is significantly influenced by the dose administered and the timing relative to feeding. Access to hay is reported to delay the time of peak plasma concentration to 18 h or longer. The bioavailability of oral phenylbutazone has been reported to be up to nearly 70%. Paste preparations may be more slowly absorbed than other preparations and yield higher residual plasma levels at 24 h after dosing, Oral phenylbutazone exhibits significant variation in the timing and magnitude of plasma levels among horses. However, after 24 hours of a single oral dose, a clear dose response relation has been reported. In this same study, after 4 days of an oral dose of 8.8 mg/kg every 12 hours, the mean peak plasma levels of phenylbutazone were 24 micrograms/ml with evidence of showed evidence of drug accumulation. In another study, blood levels of phenylbutazone administered intravenously were reported to decline with an elimination half-life of 3-10 h. The plasma kinetics of phenylbutazone were suggested to be dose dependent, with the plasma half-life increasing with the drug dose. Plasma residues of the drug at 24 h after a single intravenous dose of 2 g/450 kg average are reported to average about 0.9 microgram/ml, but considerable variation occurs. If dosing is repeated, the plasma residue accumulates to give mean residual blood levels of approximately 4.5 microgram/ml on Day 5 after 4 days of dosing. Another investigation reported that after administering 4.4 mg/kg (2g/1000lbs) intravenously for 4 days to Thoroughbred and Standardbred horses at pasture, the mean plasma concentrations of phenylbutazone increased from 0.77 microgram/ml on day 2 to 2.5 micrograms/ml on day 5. The data were reported to be consistent with one horse in 1,000 yielding a plasma level of 8.07 micrograms/ml by day 5. After administration of 8.8 mg/kg (4 g/1000 lbs) orally for 3 days, followed by 4.4 mg/kg (2 g/1000 lbs) intravenously on the 4th day to Thoroughbred and Standardbred horses at pasture, the mean plasma concentrations of phenylbutazone were 3.4 micrograms/ml on day 2 and 3.5 micrograms/ml on day 5. The range on day 5 was from 1.4 to 8.98 micrograms/ml. These data were reported to be consistent with one horse in 1000 having a plasma level of 15.8 micrograms/ml on day 5. . In a final experiment in the same report, the 8.8 mg/kg oral dose was administered for 3 days to 62 Thoroughbred horses in training. Plasma concentrations on day 5 in these horses averaged 5.3 micrograms/ml. The range was from 1.3 to 13.6 micrograms/ml. The statistical projection of these values in this report suggested that following this oral dosing schedule in racing horses about one horse in 1000 will yield a plasma level of 23.5 micrograms/ml of phenylbutazone 24 h after the last dose.

Phenylbutazone is used extensively in horses for a variety of common musculoskeletal disorders including navicular syndrome, laminitis, degenerative joint disease. The use of PBZ in performance horses is highly regulated by individual performance associations. Because PBZ may alleviate lameness in horses for several days following its use, this drug may be used to disguise lameness for the purpose of soundness examinations or for competitive purposes. PBZ appears to be less effective for visceral pain control and for endotoxemia than flunixin meglumine. An initial dose of 4.4 mg/kg every 12 hours for the first day of thcrapy is followed by 2.2 mg/kg once a day for several days. Phenylbutazone is regarded as having the most potential for toxicity of all of the NSAIDs routinely administered to horses.Due to drug accumulation from the slow excretion of oxyphenbutazone, long-term PBZ therapy for chronic conditions should be extended to every other day, with utilization of the lowest effective dose and consideration for ulcer prophylaxis and alternative analgesic approaches. Toxicity to the gastrointestinal tract is the most prominent adverse effect of PBZ therapy in horses, but PBZ also causes kidney damage from inhibiting the prostaglandins that maintain kidney blood flow and is significantly exacerbated by dehydration. Phenylbutazone competes for the same cellular binding sites as thyroid hormone. Treating horses for just 5 days causes a significant decrease in baseline thyroid hormone (T3 and T4) concentrations. Treated horses have a greater than normal response to injection with thyroid stimulating hormone. Liver disease may impair conversion of phenylbutazone to oxyphenbutazone, leading to higher free phenylbutazone blood levels and to the potential for toxicity.

Dipyrone

The pharmacology of dipyrone has not been well investigated in horses. Dipyrone is thought to act similarly to other NSAIDs by inhibiting cyclooxygenase. Dipyrone is available as a 50% solution (500 mg/ml), and can be administered IV, IM or SC to horses. Dipyrone has mild analgesic, antipyretic, and slight anti-inflammatory properties. It reportedly has antispasmodic activity on bradykinin-induced spasms of the gastrointestinal tract (spasmodic colic), but does not have the potency of flunixin meglumine for visceral pain. Dipyrone does not affect normal intestinal motility. Most veterinarians feel that other analgesic agents are more effective than dipyrone in the therapy of equine colic or pain. High doses or chronic therapy with dipyrone may result in damage to the bone marrow as manifest by abnormal blood cell production. Other adverse reactions include gastrointestinal upset, pain at the injection site, skin reactions, hemolytic anemia, tremors, and anaphylactic (allergic) reactions. It should not be administered to horses with blood or bone marrow problems. It should not be administered concurrently with acepromazine, phenylbutazone, or barbiturate anesthetics. Dipyrone is not commercially available and most veterinarians that use this medication are likely to have it compounded for use.

Flunixin Meglumine

Flunixin meglumine is a potent inhibitor of cyclooxygenase that is available in injectable, oral paste and oral granule formulations. Flunixin meglumine is rapidly absorbed following oral administration, and peak blood levels occur within 30 minutes. The onset of anti-inflammatory and analgesic action is within 2 hours and the duration of action may extend to 36 hours. As other NSAIDs, flunixin meglumine is highly protein bound. It is eliminated by the kidneys, and can be measured in urine for 48 hours following a single dose. Flunixin's pain relieving effect appears to last beyond the persistence of significant blood levels. This duration of pain relief may be due to accumulation of the drug within inflamed tissues and due to the interaction of flunixin with opiod receptors in the central nervous system in a manner similar to morphine..

Flunixin is used as an anti-inflammatory and analgesic agent in horses for a variety of conditions including; colic and other visceral pain, colitis, exertional rhabdomyolysis, endotoxemia, pleurodynia, ocular inflammation and pain, general surgery, laminitis, and other musculoskeletal disorders. Flunixin exhibits superior anti-endotoxic activity to other NSAIDs. The recommended dose is 1.1 mg/kg of body weight once daily intravenously, but higher doses and frequencies are often utilized for painful conditions such as colic. Low dose therapy with flunixin, at one quarter the label dose administered three to four times a day, has anti-endotoxic effects without masking signs of colic pain or causing toxicity. The intramuscular administration is inadvisable due to singinficant incidence of tissue reaction and necrosis. Intramuscular injections of flunixin have been associated with fatal cases of clostridial myositis. Although not all equine veterinarians agree, extremely high doses of flunixin have been proposed to mask signs of surgical colic pain. Flunixin has similar adverse effects to PBZ, but appears somewhat less toxic than PBZ in horses. High doses can result in loss of appetite, depression, and gastrointestinal tract ulcers.

Meclofenamic Acid

Meclofenamic acid is a very palatable oral granule used in horses as an analgesic and an anti-inflammatory agent for musculoskeletal conditions. This drug has not been extensively researched in veterinary medicine. Feeding prior to dosing may delay absorption of meclofenamic acid from the horse's stomach. Meclofenamic acid is typically dosed in horses at 2.2 mg/kg of body weight. Arquel is the commercially available product and it is administerd as 20 grams of granules per 1000 lb horse, once a day in the feed. Its anti-inflammatory and analgesic action can take 36-96 hours to develop. Therefore, the drug is often used, when permitted, in anticipation of joint inflammation or in preparation for a competition. Clinical efficacy can be seen for days once therapy is discontinued. Repeated daily dosing does not result in drug accumulation, making it a useful drug for chronic inflammatory conditions such as navicular disease or bone spavin. Many horses can be maintained comfortably with twice weekly dosing without side effects. This drug appears to be relatively less toxic than most of the other NSAIDs. At normal doses, some decrease in blood protein concentrations may be seen. Doses much higher than the label dose appear to be necessary to induce toxicity which may include; mouth ulcers, loss of appetite, depression, edema and weight loss.

Ketoprofen

Ketoprofen is a propionic acid derivative. Ketoprofen blocks the production of cyclooxygenase derived mediators of inflammation. Ketoprofen and its active metabolites persist in inflamed tissues at concentrations higher than those obtained in the blood. Therefore, the anti-inflammatory effects of ketoprofen are not directly related to its concentration in the blood. Ketoprofen is rapidly eliminated from the blood, therefore kidney-damaging drug accumulation does not occur. The anti-inflammatory effects of ketoprofen peak at 12 hours after a dose and last for about 24 hours. The advantages claimed for the use of ketoprofen in horses include inhibition of bradykinin and inhibition of both cyclooxygenase and lipoxygenase pathways. This anti-lipoxygenase effect is seen in laboratory studies, but has not been demonstrated in actual studies involving live horses. A purported cartilage-protective effect reported from investigations using cartilage cultures in the laboratory has not been demonstrated in the horse. Ketoprofen is recommended for musculoskeletal injuries, where a single dose provides pain relief and anti-inflammatory activity for 24 hours. Clinically in horses, ketoprofen does not appear to offer significant benefit over the use of flunixin meglumine, but appears to be less likely to cause gastrointestinal ulcers than other NSAIDs. In a small toxicity study in horses, ketoprofen produced fewer gastrointestinal lesions than treatment with flunixin meglumine or phenylbutazone. At doses many times the label dose, clinical signs of ketoprofen toxicity are similar to those seen with other NSAID toxicities.

Firocoxib (Equioxx)

This new NSAID is the first cyclooxygenase-1 (COX-1) sparing drug to be approved by the FDA for use in horses. *In vitro* studies have shown Firocoxib to be highly selective for cyclooxygenase-2 (COX-2), which is responsible for the production of inflammatory mediators. It is concurrently highly sparing of cyclooxygenase-1 (COX-1) activity, which is involved in production of prostaglandins for maintenance of physiologic functions including gastric cytoprotection, renal homeostasis, and normal platelet function. Firocoxib was restricted to use outside competition until the rule allowing its use took effect August 1, 2007. The new USEF (United States Equestrian Federation) rule lists firocoxib as a NSAID with a restrictive quantitative limit and allows for a maximum permitted concentration of 0.240 micrograms per milliliter of blood plasma. The recommendation for appropriate dose and time consideration is consistent with the manufacturer's guidelines for its use at 0.1 milligram per kilogram of body weight once daily. This dose corresponds to a 45.5 milligram dose for a 1000 lb. horse, which should be given no closer than 12 hours prior to competing. Firocoxib can be used for a period of 14 consecutive days. Per manufacturer recommendation, firocoxib should not be used in a horse in the 30 days prior to competing in a Fédération Equestre Internationale event, although a shorter interval may be more appropriate. Elimination of Firocoxib occurs primarily as the metabolite, decyclopropylmethylated metabolite in the urine. Some of the COX-2– selective anti-inflammatory agents have been reported to help ease pain in dogs but did not show disease-modifying beneficial effect. It is important to continue to focus on decreasing the progression of disease. At this time, it is unclear if that is a characteristic of the COX-2–selective anti-inflammatory agents.

Topical NSAID (Diclofenac Sodium)

Diclofenac is a nonsteroidal anti-inflammatory drug (NSAID) with analgesic properties. The phenylacetic acid NSAID diclofenac sodium is a nonselective cyclooxygenase and lipoxygenase inhibitor that is commonly used in human medicine. The safety profile of topical diclofenac has been clearly established in humans; its efficacy is equivalent or superior to that of other commonly used NSAIDs, while the risk for gastrointestinal irritation and renal toxicity is relatively low. Although there is not a diclofenac product approved for oral or parenteral administration in horses, the FDA recently approved a1% diclofenac liposomal cream formulation (Surpass [1% diclofenac sodium] Topical Anti- Inflammatory Cream, IDEXX Pharmaceuticals) for topical administration to horses for control of joint pain and inflammation associated with osteoarthritis. The drug is recommended for application in the horse by application of a five-inch (5") ribbon of SURPASS topical cream twice daily over the affected joint for up to ten days. Signs of effects include those characteristic of the NSAID group. This includes gastrointestinal and renal toxicity. Colic and weight loss and jaundice were also listed as potential adverse effects with this medication. Topical diclofenac has been cited as effective for the control of joint pain and inflammation associated with osteoarthritis. However, at least one study that investigated the anti-inflammatory efficacy of diclofenac dietilamine, applied epicutaneously at a dose rate of 0.44 mg/ kg in a model of acute arthritis in horse (using four clinical end-points and two biochemical markers) indicated a lack of pharmacological effect of this compound after epicutaneous administration. Another study was performed to evaluate the urinary and serum concentrations of diclofenac after topical administration of 1% liposomal diclofenac cream for 10 days at the labeled dose and at 2× and 4× the labeled dose. The results demonstrated the slow absorption and elimination of 1% liposomal diclofenac cream. Following 10 days of topical application of 1% diclofenac liposomal cream at 1×, 2×, and 4× the recommended label dose, diclofenac and 4-hydroxydiclofenac were present in all urine samples collected up to 72 hours after the final application. The highest urine concentrations of diclofenac occurred 6 hours after the final application of the cream. After administration of 1×, 2×, and 4× the label dose twice daily for 10 days, the decline in diclofenac and 4 hydroxydiclofenac concentrations occurred gradually over the next 3 days, with both the parent compound and the metabolite present in concentrations above the LOQ of the assay (4.0 to 8.0 ng/ml) 72 hours after the last application of each dosage regimen.

Although the clinical efficacy of diclofenac was questioned in one study, other recent work has suggested that the commercially available form of diclofenac for horses (Surpass) exhibits disease-modifying effects for osteoarthritis. Further clinical application of this formulation of diclofenac is advocated for horses that have a tendency to have swelling after hard work, especially around the fetlock joints and for routine topical management of horses with joint inflammation and/or disease. Treatment protocols for synovitis and capsulitis focus on two end points: symptom- modifying effects and disease-modifying effects. Comparison of diclofenac sodium to phenylbutazone in disease-modifying effect appears to favor diclofenac over phenylbutazone. In this comparison, a relative decrease in cartilage lesions was observed histologically in the diclofenac-treated group over the phenylbutazone treated group. Fewer side effects are likely to be encountered with topical diclofenac usage as well. It tests

DRUGS USED SPECIFICALLY FOR NAVICULAR SYNDROME (ISOXUPRINE, METRENPERONE, PENTOXFYLLINE, ASPIRIN, WARFARIN)

The use of isoxsuprine to treat navicular disease is controversial. Some studies show that horses treated with isoxsuprine hydrochloride respond favorably. Currently, there is no documented correlation between severity of lameness or radiological change of the navicular bone and and response to treatment with isoxuprine. Therefore, isoxsuprine is used empirically as a vasodilator to improve the decreased blood flow believed to occur as a part of this syndrome. Despite its widespread use, another body of research fails to show a positive response to this drug. Pharmacokinetic analysis of isoxsuprine indicates that the horse fails to absorb more than 2% of the orally administered dose. Despite this, there have been cases of positive drug tests for isoxsuprine under USEF rules. Isoxsuprine is not a permitted medication and requires a medication report and a 24 inteval prior to competition.

Metrenperone is a serotonin antagonist and thereby increases circulation. It has been used at a dose of 0.1mg/kg b.i.d. However, the drug has not been shown to be as efficacious as isoxsuprine. Another drug that is used for navicular disease is pentoxifylline, which increases RBC deformability and thus aids circulation. The drug is dosed at 4.5-7mg/kg t.i.d. Clinical trials in Canada have shown much promise. Pentoxifylline is able to increase the flexibility of red blood cells, reduce blood viscosity, and increase the blood's ability to break down blood clots. The overall effect is to make blood more liquid and to enable the red blood cells to travel deeper into tissues than they would normally be able to. This enables better oxygen delivery to tissues and improved circulation from smaller blood vessels. Aspirin is occasionally used for navicular disease in order to facilitate circulation by virtue of its anti-platelet activity.

Warfarin has been suggested for navicular syndrome. In one study, the benchmark for prolongation of the one stage prothrombin time (OSPT) to 2 to 4 seconds. The dose was initially 0.018 mg/kg, and changed by amounts of 20 per cent until the required dose was achieved. Final dose rates varied from 0.012 mg/kg to 0.75 mg/kg. Seventeen of 20 animals became sound and the remaining 3 showed a marked improvement in their gait. The mean of the periods of lameness was 9 months and the mean of the time taken to recovery one treatment was commenced was 7 weeks. Due to a narrow therapeutic window, the use of warfarin is likely to require close monitoring of coagulation and bleeding tendencies. Warfarin and PBZ compete for protein binding sites in the blood. With the administration of PBZ to a horse on warfarin therapy, the PBZ displaces some of the warfarin from protein binding sites. If the amount of protein binding of warfarin is reduced to 98%, then the concentration of free warfarin effectively doubles (to 2%) and can cause a bleeding crisis in the horse.

MUSCLE RELAXERS

Muscle spasticity may be associated with numerous clinical conditions, including trauma, myositis, muscular and ligamentous sprains and strains, vertebral conditions, tetanus, neurologic disorders, and exertional rhabdomyolysis. An increase in tonic stretch reflexes originates from the central nervous system with subsequent stimulation of descending neural tracts that leads to hyperexcitability of the motor neurons. Muscle relaxers can help alleviate muscle hyper-excitability and spasm by modifying the stretch reflex or by interference with excitation contraction coupling directly in the muscle. Centrally acting muscle relaxants act to block the interneuronal pathways in the spinal cord and reticular activating system. As a result, some drugs may also exhibit sedative effects.

Methocarbamol is a muscle relaxant that acts centrally and has a chemical structure similar to guaifenesin. Methocarbamol diminishes skeletal muscle hyperactivity while maintaining normal muscle tone. This drug effectively interrupts the transmission of abnormal impulses from hyperexcitable muscle while maintaining the normal contractile mechanism of skeletal muscle. Methocarbamol is frequently used to treat muscle spasms associated with back problems, and exertional rhabdomyolysis. Methocarbamol can be administered safely with nonsteroidal anti-inflammatory drugs, corticosteroids. An injectable formulation of methocarbamol is FDA approved for use in horses in the treatment of inflammatory and traumatic conditions of skeletal muscle in order to reduce muscle spasm and to promote muscle relaxation. The oral formulation of methocarbamol is commonly used in performance horse practice for the treatment and management of sore backs and muscle strain. It has also been prescribed preventively for horses prone to exertional rhabdomyolysis. As a CNS depressant, methocarbamol may produce sedation that can affect coordination and performance. It should not be administered with other drugs that depress the CNS. Overdosage is generally characterized by CNS depression, but salivation, weakness, and ataxia may also be seen. Although oral methocarbamol is not FDA approved, its use in the horse is a common and accepted practice. Methocarbamol is either a regulated or prohibited substance in most sanctioned competitions. It is an ARCI (Association of Racing Commissioners International) class 4 drug (therapeutic medications with less potential to affect performance than class 3 drugs). Detection times are dose related. The USEF has issued general recommendations concerning doses and timing to help competitors comply with the restrictions. The USEF drug rules may be viewed in the chart presented later in this chapter.

Dantrolene is a hydantoin derivative that is structurally and pharmacologically different from other skeletal muscle relaxants. Unlike methocarbamol, dantrolene has a direct action on muscle, and is believed to interfere with the release of calcium from the sarcoplasmic reticulum. Dantrolene has no discernible effects on respiratory and cardiac function, but may cause dizziness and sedation. In veterinary medicine, dantrolene is recommended for the treatment of malignant hyperthermia in pigs, but has been used in horses for postanesthetic myositis and exertional rhabdomyolysis. Dantrolene has also been used for the prevention of exertional rhabdomyolysis in performance horses prone to "tying up".

Phenytoin is another hydantoin derivative, primarily used as an anticonvulsant in humans. Phenytoin has been reported to be effective in some horses susceptible to exertional rhabdomyolysis. Phenytoin appears to alter the function of neurotransmitters at the neuromuscular junction, the release of calcium from the sarcoplasmic reticulum, and sodium flux at the sarcolemma. Dosages are adjusted in horses to maintain serum concentrations of 5-10 μg/mL. Though potentially effective, this drug is illegal to utilize for competitions.

CORTICOSTEROIDS

Cortisol and corticosterone are the natural body corticosteroids produced by the adrenal glands. The corticosteroids have potent anti-inflammatory activity by stimulating production of lipocortin, which inhibits phospholipase A2, the enzyme responsible for cleaving arachadonic acid from damaged cell walls. Therefore corticosteroids effectively inhibit both the lipoxygenase and cyclooxygenase pathways of inflammation. This activity blocks the production of leukotrienes as well as prostaglandins. In addition to blocking inflammatory mediators, corticosteroids also suppress white blood cell function and antibody production. This is reflected by reduction in the number of circulating white blood cells and by the white blood cell response to injured and infected tissues.

Comparison of the relative activities of the veterinary formulations of corticosteroids.

Drug	Relative Anti-inflammatory Potency	Relative Sodium-retaining Potency	Approximate Duration of Action based on Adrenal Suppression (hr)	Duration of Action (Category)
Cortisol (Hydrocortisone)	1	1	<12	Short acting
Cortisone	0.8	0.8	<12	Short acting
Prednisolone	4	0.8	12-36	Intermediate
Prednisone	4	0.8	12-36	Intermediate
Methylprednisolone	5	0-0.5	12-36	Intermediate (often regarded as drug long acting in joint)
Triamcinolone	3-5	0	24-48	Intermediate
Isoflupredone	17	0	-	Long acting (often regarded as short to intermediate in joint)
Betamethasone	25-30	0	>48	Long acting
Dexamethasone	25-30	0	>48	Long acting
Flumethasone	30	0	>48	Long acting

With acute inflammation, corticosteroids preserve the integrity of the blood vessels, reducing edema formation, and limiting the movement of white blood cells into injured tissues. In later stages of wound healing, corticosteroids reduce the proliferation of blood vessels and connective tissue, which decreases scar tissue production and slows wound healing. Although there are numerous preparations of corticosteroids available for veterinary use, they may differ significantly in their potency and duration of activity. They are commonly referred to collectively as "steroids" or "cortisone". The corticosteroids can be classified by comparing them to hydrocortisone or cortisol, the natural corticoid hormone. Feedback inhibition produced by high blood levels of either endogenous or exogenous corticosteroids is the major control of the body's release of ACTH and resultant release of endogenous corticosteroids. This activity can be used as a measure of the duration and potency of exogenously administered corticosteroids. The following tables show a comparison of the relative activities of the veterinary formulations of corticosteroids.

Relative activities of the veterinary formulations of corticosteroids.

Drug	Duration	Comparative Potency*
Hydrocortisone	8-12 hrs	1
Prednisone	12-36 hrs	4
Methylprednisone	12-36 hrs	5
Triamcinolone	12-36 hrs	5
Isoflupredone	12-36 hrs	50
Dexamethasone	32-48 hrs	30
Betamethasone	32-48 hrs	30
Flumethasone	>48 hrs	120

*Potency is determined by comparison to a cortisol a value of 1.0.

Topical Capsaicin

Capsaicin is the active chemical in hot chili peppers. Application on the equine limb is suggested to stimulate the nerve fiber to release substance P, the chemical responsible for transmitting the nervous signal for pain. Repeated application of capsaicin may act to deplete the nerve's stores of substance P, and halt the transmission of the pain signal. A number of products containing capsaicin have been developed and marketed for use in the horse (Equi-Block, Equi-Block DT, and Equi-Tite). However, there are no scientific reports to specifically support the use of these products to control pain in horses. Furthermore, the effective concentration of capsaicin and its ability to penetrate horse skin is not determined. Because these products are not marketed as drugs, there is no requirement for the manufacturer to prove clinical efficacy. An additive concern may be that if topical capsaicin is effective in alleviating pain by the mechanisms proposed, there is no presumable disease modifying properties of this drug. If this is the case, in effect, its effect would be similar to that of a local anesthesia. For certain conditions, this could facilitate severe damage induced by continued use of a horse with an injury that requires management beyond pain modification. Capsaicin may produce a painful burning and tingling sensation that could be associated with significant skin reactions. Testing for the use topical capsaisin and related blocking agents is being successfully conducted at many equine competitions using thermographic imaging and ,blood and urine testing .

Tiludronic Acid (Tildren)

'Tildren' is composed of Tiludronic acid, a bisphosphonate, a drug class with activity on bone metabolism. The main pharmacological property of Tiludronic acid is to reduce bone resorption by inhibiting the activity of osteoclast. Tiludronic acid acts as a regulator of bone remodeling in any situation involving excessive bone resorption. This regulatory effect is not associated with a negative effect of bone formation or bone mineralization at the recommended therapeutic dosage. Tiludronic acid also helps to activate the osteoblasts and to reduce the work of the osteoclasts. It exhibits anti-inflammatory effects on arthritis, mediated by interleukin-1, through inhibition of the secretion of cartilage resorbing enzymes. This property of Tiludronate may be beneficial in treating degenerative osteo-articular pathologies and may suggest that the drug exhibits osteoarthritis disease modifying properties. In addition to inhibition of the osteoclast, Tiludronate inhibits the osteoblastic synthesis of interleukin-6 and its activation of osteoclasts. The specific effects of tiludronic acid on bone resorption include binding of tiludronate, via a covalent bond, to the mineral phrase of the bone (hydroxyapatite), preferentially at the sites of bony remodeling. Acidification of the medium resulting from the initiation of the resorption process breaks the tiludronate-hydroxyapatite bond. In this way Tiludronic acid is released into the resorption cavity. The release of the Tiludronic acid leads to its penetration of the osteoclast, where it inhibits the action of the proton pump. A subsequent disruption of the cytoskeleton leads to the loss of the ruffled border and the formation of a cytotoxic ATP analogue, which causes the death of the osteoclast. Intestinal absorption of calcium is also increased in a dose dependent manner by tilduronic acid, without increasing the excretion of calcium via the urine. Tiludronic acid facilitates the binding of blood calcium to bone, by increasing the size of existing hydroxyapatite crystals or of crystals being formed. Tiludronic acid limits the release of bone calcium by the inhibition of resorption. Through these mechanisms, Tilduronic acid enhances calcium absorption, increases bone density and acts as a regulator of bone remodeling. As a consequence of its various pharmacological properties, Tiludronic acid is beneficial in the treatment of lameness where bone pathology is involved, in particular, where radiographs where osteolysis and sclerosis are present.

Tiludronic acid is reported to be helpful in the treatment of lameness associated with navicular syndrome, osteoarthritis, bone spavin and other osseous causes of lameness. It is reported to be most effective for cases with clinical signs of less than 6 months duration. Although currently unavailable in the United States, veterinarians may contact the FDA and apply to have the drug imported for specific horses by showing clinical indication for the drug in the intended recipient horse. In double-blind, placebo-controlled clinical trials for both conditions, treatment with intravenous tiludronic acid induced a clear improvement of lameness as demonstrated by long-term reduction in lameness and progressive resumption of sporting activity. A placebo-controlled clinical trial involving the treatment of back pain associated with bony lesions of the vertebral column with tiludronic acid resulted in clear improvement in back flexibility. The anti-arthritic properties of tiludronic acid have been supported by inhibitory effects on the secretion of enzymes which degrade cartilage matrix. Tiludronic acid is recommended at a dose of 0.1mg/ kg bodyweight once daily for 10 days by slow intravenous injection (10mL or 1 vial of reconstituted solution per 500kg bodyweight per day for consecutive 10 days). This drug has also been given as a single bolus intravenously and diluted in at least 1 liter of fluids. Anecdotal experience indicates a higher rate of the side effects, particularly colic, when the entire 10 day dose of the medication is given as a single bolus. This has anecdotally appeared to be particularly common when the drug is not well diluted in IV fluids. Oral administration of tilduronic acid is currently associated with and undefined bioavailability.

INTRAMUSCULAR AND INTRAVENOUS JOINT SUPPLEMENTS CHONDROPROTECTIVE DRUGS

Chondroprotective drugs are used to prevent or slow the progression of degenerative joint disease. Their effect on clinical signs of lameness is limited in comparison to that of anti-inflammatory drugs. Instead, chondroprotective drugs are utilized to facilitate chondrocyte health and function in the prevention and reduction of damage to joint cartilage that occurs from the release of enzymes and inflammatory mediators.

Hyaluronic acid or hyaluronan (HA), is a normal component of joint cartilage and fluid. It has been widely used as a treatment for joint diseases of horses and is commonly administered by intravenous administration and direct injection into the affected joint. Chemically, HA is an unsulfated glycosaminoglycan. It is produced by a membrane lining the joint capsule and is released into the joint fluid and is subsequently taken up by the joint cartilage. HA provides joint lubrication and protection of joint cartilage from the shear and compressive forces of joint motion. HA is also shown to reduce articular prostaglandin concentration and to scavenge free radicals. Other HA effects and activities are covered in the chapter on intra-articular therapies. HA concentration in inflamed joints appears to be reduced in degenerative joint disease.

Intravenous formulations of HA provide a more convenient and less invasive route of HA administration. Despite the popularity of this mode of administration of HA, when it is given intravenously, it disperses to all the joint capsules in the body. It is unclear if or how HA administered intravenously actually produced benefit to the joints. Indeed, it has been reported that intravenously administered HA does not appear to penetrate the joints at all. Rather, HA is reported to attach to anti-inflammatory receptors of the joint capsule. Through this mechanism, intravenously administered HA has been reported to exhibit more potent anti-inflammatory activity than when it is directly injected into the joint. However, if it does not enter the joints, there would be no lubrication effect when HA is administered given intravenously. Horses treated with intravenously administered HA are reported to exhibit a reduced degree of lameness compared to untreated horses. The anti-inflammatory effect of HA when given intravenously is reported to be anywhere from 2 to 7 days. Because it works well for these short periods and is a naturally occurring substance HA is often used during major USA Equestrian or FEI sanctioned competitions in place of another medication that is more likely to result in a positive drug test. Some veterinarians administer this medication frequently during competitive events. However, rules and limitations for the administration of medications should be followed as per the event regulations.

Polysulfated Glycosaminoglycan

Polysulfated glycosaminoglycan (PSGAG) is derived from an extract of cow lung and trachea. The product is a large, sulfated and charged molecule comprised of galactosamine, glucosamine, and hexuronic acid. After its administration, PSGAG binds to cartilage components. The mechanism of action of PSGAG in joints is unclear, but there are numerous studies that demonstrate a beneficial effect in damaged joints. PSGAG is believed to exhibit anti-inflammatory properties, to decrease the effect of destructive enzymes associated with joint inflammation and disease, and to stimulate normal production of hyaluronan and glycosaminoglycan. PSGAG is commonly administered to horses by either intra-articular injection of by intramuscular administration. When using the intramuscular injection, a 500 mg dose is often administered every four days for four weeks. Equine practitioners often advocate administration of additional doses at weekly or monthly intervals anecdotal benefit. Polysulfated glycosaminoglycan is related to the anti-clotting drug, heparin, and has some similar effects on blood clotting in horses. Although bleeding tendencies have been seen in people, prolonged administration of PSGAG in horses and dogs does not cause clinically apparent bleeding problems. Because of the potential for joint inflammation and infection from direct injection of the joint, many veterinary practitioners prefer the intramuscular product. Commercially available PSGAG (Adequan) is advocated for preventive or therapeutic intervention of degenerative joint disease. In several studies intramuscularly administered PSGAG was shown to penetrate and incorporate into newly produced cartilage. PSGAG works to help heal damaged cartilage. The end result is presumably a healthier joint more capable of resisting the wear and tear imposed by athletic use. There appears to be minimal anti-inflammatory effect of intramuscular PSGAG administration. Therefore, the use of such a product is more important for long term joint health and maintenance. Following the initial series of intramuscular administration, equine veterinarians often advocate continued regular dosing according to the client expectations, willingness and financial considerations. Strategic planning of the use if this drug can be helpful to control expense for the client while maximizing benefits.

"Generic" Hyaluronic Acid and Polysufated Glycosaminoglyan Type Drugs (Hycoat, Chondroprotect, Polyglycan, MAP-5, Etc)

An ever-expanding number of drugs are being produced by many companies in order to compete with Legend for the market in hyaluronic acid and with Adequan for the polysulfated glycosaminoglycan market. The vast majority of these "generic" drugs are not labeled for intravascular administration. Instead many are labeled for use in wounds to facilitate wound healing, and/or they have no supportive research in their efficacy of producing the clinical effects perceived with the 2 proprietary products, Legend and Adequan. However, there is extensive use of these "generic" products in order to facilitate more economical and more frequent administration of the same or similar compounds to horses in competition. It is imperative to recognize that this constitutes off-label use and thereby cannot be defended or justified in the eyes of a court if there should occur an otherwise untoward effect. Nonetheless, it is clear that many of these products are used extensively in equine practice with a variety of associated anecdotal reports of clinical success. Their use is not substantiated by any research or field investigation, and the response to the drug may depend on the formulation and method of production by the company that markets it.

Nutraceuticals – Chondroitin Sulfates/Glucosamines

To date, there is no significant evidence to suggest that effective absorption of nutraceuticals from the equine gut occurs in a clinically relevant manner. There has been significant debate about whether horses can absorb oral forms of joint supplementation. We have used extrapolated data from human research. Since horses are herbivores and have different GI absorption characteristics, efficacy of oral supplementation is in question until further studies can be done. Furthermore, if these products are absorbed and if the horse is capable of utilizing them, they must be combined into a very complex, large molecule in order to be effective. One cannot assume that, even if these complex molecules are included in the formulation of the nutraceutical, they are absorbed intact by the intestinal tract (without being broken down) and then reassembled into the same molecule, transported to the joints, penetrate the joint capsule and enter the joint environment to be of benefit. As supplements, nutraceutical manufacturers are not required to prove efficacy or benefit. Furthermore, the Food and Drug Administration does not regulate the formulation of glucosamine and chondroitin sulfate-containing supplements and, therefore, their purity and content are not assured. The use of products that provide certified contents from reputable sources is recommended. Despite these facts, there has been a significant increase in the popularity of using nutritional supplements to treat and prevent osteoarthritis in horses. There are numerous compounds found in the marketed products. The condroprotective neutriceuticals usually contain glucosamine salts and/or chondroitin sulfate. Cartilage cells normally synthesize glucosamine from glucose and amino acids, however they can also use externally supplied, preformed glucosamine. Regardless of the source, the cartilage cells use glucosamine to synthesize glycosaminoglycans and hyaluronan. Glucosamine also regulates cartilage synthesis of proteoglycans and collagen. Glucosamine and chondroitin sulfate are the compounds that have received the most investigation and have shown the greatest potential for benefit. Advocates of nutraceutical administration presume to believe that the compounds included in their choice formulation not only provide symptomatic relief of arthritis pain, but also help to prevent the continued degeneration of articular cartilage.

Molecularly, glucosamine is a precursor of the subunits of the cartilage matrix molecules, the proteoglycans. Laboratory studies indicate that glucosamine increases proteoglycan synthesis by chondrocytes. Glucosamine may also exhibit a number of anti-inflammatory activities. Glucosamine appears to be effective in reducing the suppressive effects of some cytokines on cartilage proteoglycan synthesis. Glucosamine has been shown to be protective against proteoglycan loss in equine cartilage and and to inhibit the synthesis and activities of degradative proteinases in equine cartilage explants. Other investigations have also demonstrated the capability of glucosamine to reduce the synthesis of matrix metallo-proteinases induced by inflammatory mediators. These effects were reported to occur at concentrations of glucosamine approaching those achieved by oral administration. Chondroitin sulfate is the principal glycosaminoglycan of aggregating proteoglycan (aggrecan). Chondroitin resembles PSGAG in structure and, though less sulfated, it appears to exhibit mechanisms of action that parallel those of PSGAG. In chondrocyte culture experiments, the chondroprotective effects of chondroitin sulfate included stimulation of proteoglycan synthesis and inhibition of matrix degrading enzymes. Chondroitin sulfate has shown protective effects on proteoglycan loss in animal models of joint inflammation.

Although there are many clinical trials involving human arthritis patients and the use of chondroitin sulfate and glucosamine, alone or in combination, many of these trials suffer from suboptimal design. There is comparatively few clinical research studies conducted on the effects of these compounds in horses. Most laboratory investigations of glucosamine and chondroitin sulfate do suggest potential favorable effects for the protection cartilage from degradation. Clinical symptomatic relief appears to be limited, particularly in advanced cases. It has been suggested that the benefit of the use of these compounds may be more for the prevention of osteoarthritis than for therapy of existing disease. These products appear to be safe and may help improve a lameness condition, but are somewhat expensive for long-term therapy.

Dimethylglyeine (DMG) and Methylsulfonylmethane (MSM)

Dimethylglycine (DMG) is also a nutriceutical product advocated for daily feeding to improving stamina and endurance by increasing oxygen utilization and improved lactic acid metabolism. Despite favorable anecdotal reports, DMG did not produce any beneficial effects on cardiorespiratory function or lactic acid production in exercising Thoroughbreds. Methylsulfonylmethane (MSM) is also a nutriceutical product suggested to be a dietary source of sulphur and a derivative of dimethylsulfoxide (DMSO), a known anti-inflammatory agent. Sulfur is a necessary component of several amino acids, therefore MSM is promoted as helping to provide the "building blocks" for normal tissues, so it is thought to have some benefit in horses with degenerative joint disease. There are no published scientific studies specifically documenting a beneficial effect from feeding MSM to horses.

Depending upon the drug administration scenario, e.g., the formulation of the drug, the dose or doses administered, the frequency of administration, the route or routes of administration, the weight of the horse or pony, the health condition of the animal, etc., it is possible that the following substances and their metabolites (byproducts) might remain detectable in the blood or urine sample of the animal for a number of days following the final administration of the substance, as follows:

anabolic steroids, e.g., boldenone and stanozolol .... 90 days
long-acting tranquilizers and psychotropics, e.g.,
fluphenazine and reserpine... 90 days
shorter-acting tranquilizers and sedatives, e.g.,
acepromazine, detomidine, and xylazine.............................. 7 days
procaine and procaine penicillin... 14 days
local anesthetics other than procaine, e.g., lidocaine
and mepivacaine.. 7 days
methylprednisolone... 14 days
corticosteroids other than methylprednisolone, e.g.,
triamcinolone and betamethasone... 7 days
nonsteroidal anti-inflammatory drugs, e.g.,
phenylbutazone and flunixin... 7 days
antihistamines, e.g., cyproheptadine and pyrilamine.............. 7 days
respiratory drugs, e.g., albuterol.. 7 days

isoxsuprine.. 21 days

Any other drug or medication call (800) 633-2472 and ask.

By following the above guidelines, it will the chances of positive drug testing will be minimized. For forbidden substances; however all trainers, owners, and exhibitors are cautioned that the foregoing are only general guidelines, and it is the trainer's responsibility to see to it that conditions prevail for full compliance with all USEF rules.

2007 USEF Drug Withdrawal Guidelines

Medication Generic Name	Medication Trade Name	Max Dosage per pound of Body Weight	Latest Administration Hour Prior to Competition	Administration Method (single dose per 24 hours unless specified otherwise)
Dexamethasone	Azium	2.0 mg/100Lb (20 mg/1000Lb) or 0.5 mg/100Lb (5.0 mg/1000Lb) or 1.0 mg/100LB (10 mg/1000Lb)	>12 hours >6 hours >6 hours	IV, IM,PO
Diclofenac	Surpass	5 inch ribbon, ½ inch thick, one site	>12 hours	Topical, 2 doses each day 12 hours apart
Firocoxib	Equioxx	0.1 mg/kg (0.0455 mg/Lb) (45.5 mg/1000Lb)	>12 hours	Oral
Phenylbutazone ("bute") *	Butazolidin	2.0 mg/Lb (2.0 grams/1000Lb) or 1.0 mg/Lb (1.0 grams/1000Lb)	>12 hours AM and PM feed	Oral, IV Oral, 2 doses each day,12 hours apart
Flunixin meglumine *	Banamine	0.5 mg/Lb (500 mg/1000Lb)	>12 hours	Oral, IV
Ketoprofen	Ketofen	1.0 mg/Lb (1.0 gram/1000Lb)	>4 hours but >6 hours recommended	IV
Meclofenamic acid	Arquel	0.5 mg/Lb (500 mg/1000Lb)		Oral, 2 doses each day, 12 hours apart
Naproxen	Naprosyn	4.0 mg/Lb (4.0 grams/1000Lb)	>12 hours	Oral
Eltenac Not yet approved	Telzenac	0.25 mg/Lb (250 mg/1000Lb)	12 hours	IV
Methocarbamol	Robaxin	5.0 mg/Lb (5.0 grams/1000Lb)	>6 hours	Oral, IV 2 doses each day, 12 hours apart

REST/ REDUCTION IN EXERCISE INTENSITY

Long before veterinary medications and interventions existed, there was rest. Indeed the significance of rest and reduced exercise intensity in facilitating recovery from an acute injury or an exacerbation of a chronic condition cannot be overstated. For minor injuries or lameness, rest or controlled exercise may be the management of choice. Numerous conditions also benefit from continuous controlled exercise ranging from muscle disorders to navicular disease. The prescription of rest and/or controlled exercise intensity does not eliminate the need for a specific diagnosis. Conditions expected to respond adequately to rest or reduced exercise need to be specifically identified in order to prevent danger of re-injury and to promote satisfactory recovery. Frequently, other medical and/or procedural interventions may also be employed with controlled exercise in order to facilitate treatment response and to minimize the amount of time the horse is out of competition. Following the period of rest or reduced exercise, the horse will be returning to the same level of exercise that caused the initial problem. The sustained return to competition after an injury may itself require regular controlled exercise capable of sustaining the level of fitness and flexibility necessary to help prevent recurrence of the condition.

ICE/ HYDROTHERAPY/SUPPORT WRAPS

Supportive wraps and ice therapy are old standbys that are very helpful and under-recognized as therapeutic interventions. Horses that tend to fill in the limbs after exercise, or horses that have chronic leg conditions may benefit from regular therapy by standing in ice water or by hosing or other hydrotherapy before and/or after exercise. These may include ice and cold-compression boots that can control the inflammation on a daily basis. Further information pertaining to cold therapy is presented in the physiotherapy section of this chapter. The work intensity and schedule may need to be modified if ice/hydrotherapy and support wraps are being used to manage or treat a specific condition. Support wraps on the limbs may be important for overnight control of limb swelling. For horses with chronic joint conditions, a concurrent regimen of intravenous hyaluronic acid and intramuscular polysulfated glycosaminoglycan may also be warranted. By combining these management practices, one may be able to control joint and other conditions in horses that need to return to their previous work schedule or continue their exercise programs with chronic conditions.

Leg Sweats/ Poultice

Although sweat bandages are effective, the science of how and why they work still isn't precisely understood. Presumably, the purpose of a leg sweat is to generate heat which may help dilate vessels and increase blood flow or the heat may be generated by the dilation of the blood vessels and increased blood flow. Sweat bandages also provide external pressure to the limb and provide support. Regardless of the mechanism, the combined effect is believed to be the dissipation of excess fluid from the injury site and the reduction of inflammation. While sweat bandages are useful in reducing swelling, they are not recommended for recent injuries or those that include open wounds. Leg sweats can be irritating to the skin. Leg sweats are applied to the leg, covered with lightweight plastic wrap, and then bandaged over the plastic wrap with a regular support wrap. Homemade leg sweats are commonly used and these leg sweats commonly include one or a combination of the following ingredients; dimethylsulfoxide, nitrofuracin ointment or liquid, mineral oil, petroleum jelly, glycerine or glycerol. Many of these ingredients are believed to help deliver and subsequently increase the local concentration of the active medication. .

A poultice is generally a safe, non-irritating substance that is applied to the limb for its osmotic properties. A poultice does not induce the heat and vessel dilation that a sweat does. Rather, the poultice acts to draw edema out of the leg presumably by an osmotic action. Poultice wraps are commonly utilized following strenuous exercise in order to help prevent limb swelling, or they may be applied in order to help remove excess lower limb edema. Many commercially available brands of equine leg poultice are available. Selection of a product is primarily based on personal preference.

Proper Bandaging Techniques

It is essential to use proper techniques when applying a sweat bandage. Applied incorrectly, the bandage will not only fail to do its job, it can cause discomfort, restrict blood flow and potentially damage tendons and other tissue. A "bandage bow" due to an improperly placed leg bandage results in edema of the limb, and usually over the flexor tendons.. Generally speaking, this terminology is misleading because there is no true tendon damage that occurs with a bandage bow and the visible swelling is usually a manifestation of peritendinous edema. Appropriate padding is essential for protecting limbs and requires the use of good bandaging material such as a fleece bandage or a heavy 'quilted" bandage. Even pressure during wrapping is important when applying the external bandage to the padding wrap. It is important to leave approximately ½ to 1 inch of the padding wrap exposed at the top and bottom of the bandage to ensure that the external bandage is not or will not be in direct contact with the limb. As a convention, many horsemen prefer a specific wrapping direction. The direction of the wrap is considered to be correct when the bandages are begun on the inside of the limb and the wrapping direction is forward towards the head of the horse. This means a counter-clockwise wrap on the left side of the horse and a clockwise wrap on the right side of the horse. Physiologically, the direction of the wrap is probably irrelevant, but horsemen can be very particular and critical about this.

Internal Blister

An internal blister is a counter irritant that is injected into a tissue in order to induce inflammation and to produce a response in the tissue that results in increased blood flow and possibly scarring. For some applications, internal blistering is a form of sclerotherapy that results in a "tightening" of the injected tissue. The solutions utilized for internal blistering are by nature highly irritating. Great care must be utilized in selection of the indications and sites for an internal blister. The most common application of the use of an internal blister in performance horse practice appears to be the blister of the patellar ligaments in horses that subluxate their patellas despite regular exercise and strength of the quadriceps muscles. Frequently the distal quadriceps muscles are concurrently blistered with the patellar ligaments. The most commonly used solutions for internal blister are iodine in almond oil. At one time, there was a commercially available 2% iodine in almond oil or peanut oil. Other solutions that have been used in the past included DMSO, blood and Biotropina (an immunostimulant). These solutions are not commercially produced and most performance horse veterinarians have the solutions made by compounding pharmacies. In the past, an internal blister was more commonly used to treat splints and high suspensory injuries. This practice led to some severe complications and these applications do not seem to be as popular as they once were. Following an internal blister, horses are generally exercised immediately and regularly several times a day. This practice helps to reduce the stiffness and swelling that occur following the procedure. Clinical response to the blister is often recognized in 1 to 2 weeks following the procedure. Internal blisters are much less commonly utilized today for less irritating practices such as prolotherapy. When an internal blister is utilized, it is most often for stifle laxity.

Prolotherapy (Regenerative Injection Therapy, RIT)

Prolotherapy (proliferative therapy), also known as ligament reconstructive therapy, is a recognized orthopedic procedure that presumably stimulates the body's natural healing processes to strengthen joints weakened by injury or arthritis. The premise behind prolotherapy is similar to that of an internal blister, however, prolotherapy is usually executed with less caustic compounds and usually produces a milder form of counter-irritation and inflammation. Because of its less irritating and offensive results, and therefore its potentially wider acceptance, the application of prolotherapy to equine therapeutics may be significantly more extensive than that of the internal blister. Joints weakened when ligaments and tendons are stretched, torn, or fragmented may become hypermobile and painful. Prolotherapy may augment or even replace some traditional approaches with anti-inflammatory drugs and surgery that may fail to stabilize the joint and to relieve associated long-term pain. The utilization of prolotherapy directly addresses the cause of instability in helping to repair the weakened structures and resulting in stabilization of the joint. When precisely injected into the site of pain or injury, prolotherapy creates a mild, controlled inflammation which facilitates sclerosis of tendon, ligament fibers, or other tissue, resulting in a strengthening of the weakened structure. Multiple treatments are often required. Solutions utilized for prolotherapy may contain dextrose, calcium, phenol or a combination. Prolotherapy may be used to treat joint hypermobility, which causes excess movement. Other proposed applications of prolotherapy have included; arthritis, hip laxity and pain, cruciate injury, neck pain, back pain, spinal stenosis, disc disease, chronic tendonitis, partially torn tendons, ligaments and cartilage injuries.As a distinction from an internal blister, follow-up management of prolotherapy does not require rigorous physical activity, making prolotherapy, in combination with intra-articular therapy, a viable option.

MESOTHERAPY

Mesotherapy is a treatment that stimulates the tissues that have developed from the embryonic mesoderm. Though there is no “mesoderm layer” of the skin, the cells of the embryonic mesoderm do develop into dermis and hypodermis, fatty tissues, and the musculoskeletal system. Thus, with mesotherapy, one is not "injecting into the mesoderm," rather one is injecting into those structures that have arisen from mesoderm. Mesotherapy appears to be a novel technique to administer medicines local to the pathology using the skin acts as a natural time-release system. A proposed mechanism of action of mesotherapy is that solutions injected intracutaneously remain in the area longer than they would by deeper injection because they are slower to be cleared by general circulation. It is proposed that these solutions injected superficially continually penetrate into the deeper tissues. Mesotherapy is first and foremost considered to be a pain and sports medicine modality. Mesotherapy is of particular interest to clinicians due to its safety, tolerability to patients, cost-effectiveness, and apparent efficacy. Mesotherapists believe that, by increasing microcirculation of localized tissue beds, the elimination of metabolic waste is facilitated, and there is an increase in the delivery of the mesotherapeutic solution and oxygen. Alternatively, another hypothesis of the mechanism of action is the “gate-theory” of central nervous system (CNS) pain recognition. In this hypothesis, the CNS recognition of threshold of pain is altered following overwhelming peripheral nervous system stimulation proposed to follow mesotherapy. .

Compounds included in human mesotherapy solutions are diverse. Local anesthetics are used in the vast majority of mesotherapy protocols. Either lidocaine 1% or procaine 1%, without epinephrine is used. Local anesthetics are used for their anesthetic properties that are believed to be longer-acting when injected mesotherapeutically. As is taught by the French Society of Mesotherapy, lidocaine is generally indicated for treatment of acute conditions, while procaine is indicated for chronic conditions because of its additional vasodilatory properties. Drug testing in horses will significantly limit the use of procaine and lidocaine. Mesotherapists commonly use the vasodilatory medication buflomedil when treating pain. Buflomedil is not available in the US. Pentoxifylline (Trental), also commonly used in France, is an FDA-approved medication that is not a true vasodilator, but may be used in place of buflomedil. Pentoxifylline's on-label use is for the treatment of intermittent claudication, and it improves microcirculation by decreasing the blood's viscosity and by improving erythrocyte flexibility. Pentoxifylline has been shown to increase leukocyte deformability and inhibit neutrophil adhesion and activation. Tissue oxygen levels have been shown to significantly increase with therapeutic doses of pentoxifylline in patients with peripheral arterial disease. Reportedly, by injecting pentoxifylline mesotherapeutically, pentoxifylline exhibits antinociceptive activities. It is a tumor necrosis factor-alpha and interleukin-1-beta antagonist, and it has been shown to be an interleukin-1-alpha receptor agonist, limiting inflammatory hyperalgesia. Local administration of pentoxifylline is reported to cause inhibition of proinflammatory cytokine synthesis and antagonizes hyperalgesia in formalin-injected rats. The use of salmon calcitonin (sCT) for the treatment of a broad spectrum of chronic pain disorders is also proposed. sCT is best known as an anti-osteoporotic agent administered as a nasal spray, but its analgesic effects in the treatment of acute osteoporotic fracture has been well-documented. The mechanisms of analgesic action of sCT are believed to be multifactorial. An anti-inflammatory action has been suggested.

Studies in animals and in humans demonstrate that in some, but not all, cases, calcitonin increases plasma beta-endorphin levels. It is proposed that specific binding sites may be present for salmon calcitonin in the brain. While the use of sCT appears safe, it is not without risk of side effect or adverse reaction. Nausea without vomiting and mild local inflammatory reactions at the site of injection is reported in approximately ten percent of patients receiving sCT, and transient severe nausea and vomiting occurs in approximately one in 300 patients. Flushing of face or hands, skin rashes, nocturia, pruritus has also been reported. Administration of sCT has been reported in isolated cases to cause hypersensitivity reactions.

Mesotherapy is reported to be beneficial in the treatment of neck and chronic thoracic back pain due to arthritis, spinal stenosis, and sprain/strain not adequately controlled with conventional methods, degenerative arthritic pain, and various soft tissue musculoskeletal pain. Mesotherapy has been shown to be helpful in a variety of commonly seen sports medicine conditions. In human patients, the following protocol has been proposed for the use of ingredients that are safe, effective, and readily available internationally:

- 50IU salmon calcitonin
- 1cc Pentoxifylline 20mg/mL
- 1cc lidocaine 2%
- 0.5cc multivitamin (optional – available as a "meso-multi" from a number of US compounding pharmacies).

The mesotherapy injections involve extremely small needles that penetrate the interdermal layer of the skin only a very small depth, which is typically four to six millimeters. The number of treatments needed depends on many variables including the condition, the abnormal physiology causing the condition, as well as the chronicity of the problem. A minimum of one to two sessions of mesotherapy is performed generally to assess the horse's response. Mesotherapy is effective for a multitude of conditions because it helps reverse the physiology of that condition, and stop the pain spasm cycle. In equine practice, mesotherapy has been utilized to treat chronic neck and back pain and degenerative arthritis of the back and cervical vertebrae (neck). The following formulation has been proposed for use in the horse:

- Mesotherapy solution: 15cc Carbocaine, 3cc Flumethasone, 2 vials (6cc) Traumeel, Lactated Ringers solution.
- Mesotherapy Supplies: 2 x 60cc syringes, 1 x 30 extension set, 1 multi-injector 5 needles. Multi-injectors and needles available from: MESORAM (California) phone (909) 593-8569 Fax (909) 593-0739

Traumeel available from: Heel Biotherapeutics (800) 621-7644 Ext. 2947.

An alternative veterinarycombination includes Sarapin, Traumeel and a low dose of a short-acting corticosteroid in order to provide the desired effect with minimal side effects. Long acting steroid products (i.e., Depomedrol) has been associated with white hair growth in the area treated.

ACUPUNCTURE

Acupuncture may be defined as the stimulation of specific predetermined points on the body to achieve a therapeutic or homeostatic effect. Essentially, acupuncture stimulates various sensory receptors (pain, thermal, pressure, and touch) which subsequently stimulate sensory afferent nerves and transmit the signal through the central nervous system to the hypothalamic-pituitary system. Various neurotransmitters and neurohormones are then released and have their subsequent effects throughout the body.

There are numerous techniques used to stimulate acupuncture points. The following modes of stimulation may be employed in equine acupuncture: dry needle stimulation, electroacupuncture, aquapuncture, moxibustion, laser stimulation, gold implants, and acupressure. Each method has its indications and limitations. Detailed descriptions of these techniques are described by in acupuncture texts. Acupuncture point selection is based on locating points on the body where stimulation will produce a beneficial change in the central nervous system by modulating ongoing physiologic activity. The exact location of equine acupuncture points has been debated over the past two decades. Some veterinarians base their acupoint location on the traditional Chinese equine acupuncture maps. The Chinese did not recognize meridians on nonhuman animals, but rather had points named based on their anatomical location or their function. Other veterinarians who received their training through the International Veterinary Acupuncture Society base their equine acupuncture point location on the transpositional method. This method extrapolates and transposes human acupuncture meridians to the equine, adjusting point location to equine anatomy. Currently, this is the most accepted approach. The number of treatments required depends upon the condition treated and the chronicity of the problem.

Acupuncture has been utilized as both a diagnostic aid as an adjunct to conventional lameness examination and in therapeutic application. Acupuncture diagnosis is based on the level of sensitivity upon palpation of particular acupoints that have been found to correspond diagnostically with specific conditions. Many of the diagnostic acupoints are located lateral to the dorsal midline between the longissimus and iliocostalis muscles. In addition, there are diagnostic points that are referred to as trigger points, knots or tight bands in a muscle. For instance, a triceps trigger point is reported to be sensitive to palpation with lower forelimb lameness. It may not indicate the exact location of the lameness or its etiology, but it is believed to indicate when something is reactive in a specific region. Each diagnostic acupuncture point may have four or more meanings, depending on which other points are determined to be reactive on the acupuncture examination. For instance, sensitivity on acupoints along the bladder meridian, lateral to the dorsal midline along the back, may indicate that there is a hindlimb lameness related to the stifle or hock, or that there is a primary back problem related to the saddle fit, rider, or a conformational problem. The combination of reactive points often times will assist the diagnosis and aid in localization of the cause of the problem. Often times one may localize lower limb lameness along with a back problem. Acupoint diagnosis is reported to be potentially helpful in determining which problem occurred first. Acupuncture diagnosis may be an adjunct to the equine lameness exam in addition to flexion tests, diagnostic nerve blocks, radiographs, ultrasound, and other imaging modalities. In human medicine, they musculoskeletal pain is often reported to be accompanied by muscle shortening in peripheral and paraspinal muscles due to spasms and contractures. Secondary trigger points and autonomic manifestations of neuropathies are reported to occur with chronic musculoskeletal pain. Patterns of trigger points distant from the primary problem, compensating for the primary musculoskeletal problem, may also be found. These patterns are also reportedly evident in equine acupuncture lameness exams.

Acupuncture is also used successfully in the treatment of various equine musculoskeletal conditions either as a primary treatment or as an adjunct to conventional veterinary therapeutic techniques. For instance, one may diagnose a primary hock problem and it may be treated with an intra-articular injection. However, it may not completely resolve the entire complaint. There may be secondary compensation and subsequent patterns of trigger points in the back or neck that remain unresolved. Acupuncture therapy may then be successfully used to treat the secondary manifestations of the primary hock problem. Acupuncture has been reported to be successful for the treatment of numerous causes of equine lameness including chronic back problems, hock or stifle problems, laminitis, navicular disease as well as various soft tissue injuries. Neurologic conditions that are reported to potentially respond to acupuncture include facial nerve, sciatic nerve, and radial nerve paralysis. Referral to an equine acupuncturist is recommendable if the primary examining veterinarian does not have appropriate training in equine acupuncture. Acupuncturists may work along with the primary veterinarian in challenging lameness cases. Acupuncture offers an additional approach to diagnostic and therapeutic dilemmas that may not produce diagnosis or therapeutic solutions based on conventional western medicine.

Chiropractic Therapy

Equine chiropractic therapy has been utilized for the diagnosis, treatment, and potential prevention of select musculoskeletal disorders in horses. Although limited research has been done to evaluate the clinical effectiveness of chiropractic manipulations in horses, equine chiropractic therapy has become well accepted and often requested by clients for its perceived preventive and therapeutic effects. Chiropractic therapy utilizes controlled forces which are applied to specific articulations or anatomic regions that are suggested to induce therapeutic response by manipulating joint structures, muscle function, and neurologic reflexes.

The concepts of joint dysfunction relative to chiropractic intervention are reported to be altered articular neurophysiology, biochemical alterations, joint capsule pathology, and articular degeneration. Vertebral segment dysfunction has been described as asymmetric or loss of normal joint motion, alteration of point tenderness or diminished pain threshold to pressure in the paraspinal tissues and/or osseous structures, abnormal paraspinal muscle tension, and visual or palpation findings indicative of active inflammation or tissue texture abnormalities that include edema, fibrosis, hyperemia, or altered temperature. Altered mechanical and biochemical processes are believed to influence the neuromusculoskeletal system by producing altered joint mobility, altered articular neurophysiology and pain sensation characterized by inhibition or facilitation, altered muscle function indicated by hypertonicity, or atrophy, connective tissue changes such as fibrosis, and vascular alterations such as ischemia, and hyperemia. Alterations in articular neurophysiology from mechanical or chemical injuries are believed to affect both mechanoreceptor and nociceptor function through increased joint capsule tension and nerve ending hypersensitivity. Mechanoreceptor stimulation induces reflex paraspinal musculature hypertonicity and altered local and systemic neurologic reflexes. Nociceptor stimulation reportedly results in a reduced threshold to pain, sustained afferent stimulation (facilitation), reflex paraspinal musculature hypertonicity, and abnormal neurologic reflexes.

Back problems appear to be common in performance horses. However, the etiology of back problems in the horse is often unclear. The primary cause of a back problem may be due to an appendicular problem or to the vertebral column as the primary cause of a clinical problem. A sore back is therefore regarded as an indication for a complete lameness examination. Chiropractic conditions in performance horses usually have a history of a traumatic event or injury related to overexertion. Trauma may occur as a single event inducing "macrotrauma" such rearing and flipping, or falling over a jump. Chronic, overuse injuries (microtrauma) are believed to occur due to things such as poor saddle fit, improper riding, inadequate shoeing, or faulty conformation. Long periods of confinement, inconsistent training programs, overuse syndromes, or stresses and strains related to athletic activities may also predispose horses to musculoskeletal injuries and reduced performance. Older horses, like elderly humans, are susceptible to loss of vertebral column flexibility, joint degeneration, and loss of muscle strength.

With chiropractic intervention, the goal of treatment is to restore normal joint motion, stimulate neurologic reflexes, and to reduce pain and muscle hypertonicity. During a successful adjustment, a 'release' or movement of the restricted articulation may often be palpable. An audible 'popping' sound may also be heard during treatment as the applied force overcomes the elastic barrier of joint resistance. Rapid articular separation is said to produce cavitation of the synovial fluid. A second attempt to "release", or recavitate the joint, will be unsuccessful and potentially painful until the intra-articular gas has been reabsorbed (the refractory period). Chiropractic techniques utilize controlled force applied to a specific anatomical region or osseous structure in order to restore joint motion and reduce pain. The applied thrust is believed to influence both mechanoreceptor and nociceptor function through mechanical and biological mechanisms. The 'therapeutic dosage' of chiropractic adjustment is controlled by the number of vertebral levels adjusted, the amplitude of the applied force, and the frequency of treatment. Some research has shown that such forces applied to vertebral segments do induce substantial vertebral motion, usually beyond the normal range of segmental motion that occurs during locomotion. Horses receiving chiropractic manipulation need to be relaxed in order for the therapy to induce the desired effect to the vertebral segments. Chiropractic therapy is frequently employed with concurrent massage, physiotherapy modalities, and stretching or strengthening exercises in order to facilitate soft tissue rehabilitation and to restore vertebral joint motion. Other prescribed interventions may include an alteration in training frequency or activity, corrective shoeing and changes in tack. Repetitive use disorders have been suggested to potentially benefit from cross-training activity. Practitioners have anecdotally reported synergistic therapeutic benefit by the combination of chiropractic intervention and acupuncture or other holistic modalities.

An immediate reduction in pain and an increase in segmental vertebral motion is often recognized in response to chiropractic manipulation. Conditions with an acute onset often appear to respond rapidly, whereas chronic conditions usually require long-term intervention. Chiropractic therapy is a conservative modality that may be best utilized repetitively over time in both therapeutic and preventive applications. Post-adjustment recommendations for horses in regular training includes stall rest or pasture turnout for one day, followed by return to normal work the following day. If stiffness or soreness is detected following adjustment, an additional day of rest usually prescribed. If the horse continues to exhibit discomfort beyond this time, re-examination and, if necessary, referral for further treatment is recommended. Adverse effects of chiropractic manipulation may include transient stiffness or worsening of the clinical signs. Adverse response to chiropractic adjustment is uncommon, but may occur immediately or with insidious onset over the next 6 to 12 hours. The harmful effects from improperly applied manipulation may include permanent articular damage, torn ligaments, injured muscles, luxated joints, fractures, or paralysis.

Chiropractic therapy may be used to help manage the muscular, articular, and neurologic components of select musculoskeletal injuries in performance horses. Musculoskeletal conditions that are chronic or recurring, not readily diagnosed, or are not responding to conventional veterinary care may be indicators that chiropractic consultation may be helpful. Chiropractic care is usually contraindicated in the acute stages of soft tissue injury. However, as the soft tissue injury heals, chiropractic intervention may help restore normal joint motion. Chiropractic is generally not indicated for management of structural vertebral defects. Severe osseous changes such as joint subluxation, luxation, or fractures are often contraindications for chiropractic. However, functional defects, such as unilateral paraspinal muscle contraction or joint restrictions are likely to be amendable to chiropractic intervention. Chiropractic care may help provide symptomatic relief in early degenerative joint disease if the condition is related to joint hypomobility. Cervical myelopathy occurs due to both structural and functional disorders in the cervical vertebrae. Chiropractic therapy is contraindicated for this condition. Chiropractic therapy is likely to be more effective in the early stages of a condition or when it is used to manage and/or prevent conditions with regularity. Chiropractic therapy is not recommended for treatment of fractures, infections, neoplasia, metabolic disorders or joint disorders of a nature other than mechanical dysfunction. Acute sprains or strains, significant degenerative joint disease and spinous processes impingment are contraindications for chiropractic adjustment. Neurologic conditions should be fully evaluated in order to assess the potential risk and benefit of chiropractic intevention. Chiropractic therapy may help facilitate rehabilitation of selected post-surgical or medical conditions by helping restore normal musculoskeletal function.

Digital Neurectomy

A digital neurectomy is a surgical procedure involving transaction of the posterior digital nerve supplying primarily heel area of the equine foot. The procedure is generally considered to be a salvage procedure and not recommended until all other treatment option have been exhausted. Digital neurectomy produces loss of sensation to the area supplied by the transected nerve. Although this is effective for amelioration of chronic pain, the loss of sensation also imparts certain risks to the horse as a result of the procedure. Digital neurectomy is probably most commonly utilized to control heel pain in the horse as a result of navicular syndrome. However, any chronic and uncontrolled cause of pain that localizes to the heel of the foot may be considered a potential indication for this procedure. Although this intervention may be effective for control of chronic heel pain, there are significant complications that can occur secondary to this procedure. With loss of sensation of the heel, a rupture of the deep flexor tendon appears to be a significant risk following a digital neurectomy. Furthermore, the formation of a painful neuroma can occur following the procedure. Finally, after some undefined period of time, some horses appear to regain sensation to a certain extent, requiring a repeat of the surgical procedure. Digital neurectomies have often been done under general anesthesia, but a technique for this procedure in the standing horse has been described.

Radiofrequency Therapy (Radio Frequency Treatment)

This therapy is taken from human medicine and has been modified for use in horses by the author (MSR). Radiofrequency therapy (RF) utilizes radio frequency waves to essentially anesthetize an area by its effect on any peripheral nerve that inervates the area associated with pain. However, unlike a neurectomy that also produces complete loss of sensation of the region supplied by the transected nerve, radiofrequency therapy preserves neural sensation. The theory is that pain signals are believed to be blocked if sensory afferent neurons are sufficiently stimulated. The application of heat, or other stimulation, to an injured part might sufficiently overload the pain transmission with a preponderance of sensory input from thermoreceptors. The true mechanism of this selective effect remains unclear and initial experiments indicated that small delta and unmyelinated C fibers were preferentially destroyed by RF. Later experiments, however, showed that RF did not differentiate between nerve fibers. Despite conflicting study results, the theory of fiber selectivity remains popular as it is still unknown why pain transmission is blocked but motor transmission is unimpeded. Although this theory has been suggested, no definitive evidence exits. Radiofrequency therapy is less invasive than neurectomy, and is performed in the standing horse with sedation, local anesthesia and two small incisions. Radiofrequency therapy is therefore a safer and less invasive alternative to digital neurectomy in select cases. Radiofrequency therapy may also be used for treatment of soft tissue injuries.

Plantar Fasciotomy and Neurectomy of the Deep Branch of the Lateral Plantar Nerve

Because lameness often persists following prolonged rest and exercise restriction as the primary means to manage proximal suspensory desmitis, surgical fasciotomy has been utilized to address chronic proximal suspensory desmitis of the hindlimb. Fasciotomy is based on the premise that decompression and reduction of compartment syndrome that affects the nerve supply of the suspensory ligament contributes significantly to persistent lameness. Because nerve damage caused by entrapment and compartment syndrome may be permanent, fasciotomy alone may not provide adequate resolution to the lameness. Response to fasciotomy is likely to be improved with concurrent neurectomy of the deep branch of the lateral plantar nerve. Because the sensory and motor innnervation of the suspensory ligament is supplied by the deep branch of the lateral plantar nerve, neurectomy of a portion of this nerve is associated with improvement in lameness due to chronic proximal suspensory desmitis. Due to the resultant anesthesia of the area, reinjury and/or complete rupture of the suspensory ligament may occur with minimal clinical signs..

EXTRACORPOREAL SHOCK WAVE THERAPY (ESWT)

Over the past decade, a growing number of veterinarians are utilizing extracorporeal shockwave therapy to therapeutically address soft tissue and osseous conditions in horses. Equine shock wave therapy transmits positive pressure acoustic waves to focus on target structures at various depths and energy levels depending upon the injury being treated. The mechanism of action of shockwave therapy is unclear may but be described "controlled re-injury" and analgesia may be produced by nerve injury, altered pain perception by the central nervous system, altered intraosseous pressure, stabilization of a joint by strengthening of articular and periarticular soft tissues and/or reduction in subchondral bone edema. Some horses may experience the analgesic effect of ESWT immediately following the procedure. The duration of the analgesia provided is at least partly dependent on the condition being treated and the idiosyncratic response of the horse being treated. An analgesic effect lasting for 4 days following ESWT has been described. Beyond analgesia, a therapeutic effect of ESWT has been proposed. This effect is controversial and has yet to be proven. Nonetheless, ESWT has been reported to enhance the rate of bone healing. ESWT has also been suggested to enhance the rate of tendon and ligament healing. In addition to speeding up healing time, shockwave therapy has also been proposed to induce comparatively superior healing results to treatment of the same injury with of rest alone. ESWT is recommended for horses suffering from chronic pain and lameness, who have failed to respond to conservative treatment for a period of at least three months. In particular, problems caused by degenerative or acute processes in tendons and superficial bones are appropriate consideration for treatment using ESWT. One of the most frequently treated injuries is an injury to the proximal suspensory ligament. Following shockwave therapy of the high suspensory injury, the likelihood of returning to full function has been reported to be significantly improved. Shockwave therapy is commonly applied to the equine foot for management of specifically diagnosed heel pain. ESWT is also being used to treat stifle, back and pelvic problems. Depending upon the specific problem, dramatic responses have been reported. Shockwave therapy is usually performed on an outpatient basis. Horses are often sedated for the procedure and may require application of a twitch. Treatment usually takes lasts 10 to 15 minutes. Treatment protocols vary depending upon the specific injury. Anywhere from one to four treatment sessions are conducted. If more than one treatment is prescribed, the treatments are usually timed at a minimum of 14 days intervals. ESWT is not an appropriate treatment for all conditions causing pain in the horse. Even with excellent case selection, a number of horses with conditions expected to respond to shockwave therapy may fail to respond. However, ESWT may help avoid surgery by providing another non-invasive treatment option for appropriate of soft tissue and osseous disorders.

Stem Cell Therapy / Bone Marrow Therapy

Stem cells are immature, vigorous cells that mature into any of the hundreds of various body cell types--nerve, blood, heart, muscle, fat, bone, cartilage, etc. The perception of stem cells is often linked to the understanding of cells derived from an embryo that exhibit the ability to develop into many different types of body tissue. However, stem cells can be harvested from tissue other than embryonic tissue, including; bone marrow, fat, and umbilical cord blood. In fact, stem cells derived from tissue other than embryonic tissue are better suited for use in equine stem cell therapy of damaged tissue, and horses tend to reject embryonic stem cells. Cells harvested from the patient's own bone marrow are also showing great promise for several reasons. First, there is no risk of tissue rejection with autologous bone marrow derived stem cells. Many studies coming indicate that the adult mesenchymal stem cell (from which arises connective tissues of the body, blood vessels, and lymphatic vessels) in the human has tremendous plasticity. Bone marrow also contains fibronectin (which aids cell migration through the area of injection) and growth factors (which enhance healing). Bone marrow stem cells provide very quick pain relief, as has been seen in the human application of this intervention. Stem cells are adaptable and capable of being manipulated into becoming different types of cells. After harvesting and concentrating the stem cells in a laboratory, the stem cells and bone marrow are transferred into the damaged ligament or tendon, where they reproduce into normal, healthy tissue, improving healing and stability of the injured or diseased area. In the process, they also reduce inflammation and relieve pain. When manipulated stem cells are injected into the injured site, they grow into normal or near-normal tissue. The advantage to stem cell therapy is the quality of healing that can be obtained in the implanted tissue

A current technique is to concentrate the native stem cell population in bone marrow at the time of harvesting, then inject them along with bone marrow into the damaged ligament or tendon. In addition to bone marrow, fat is another viable source of stem cells. The cells are harvested from the tail head of the patient horse, then sent to Vet-Stem, the only commercially available laboratory in the United States that extracts the stem cells from fat. The sample is then sent back for use usually in 48 hours. The short turnaround time allows the cells to be injected soon after the initial injury. Another study of using stem cells for tendon repair found improved healing with fat-derived stem cells. The researchers found the stem cell treated lesions exhibited reduced inflammation, improved collagen fiber uniformity, higher tendon healing scores. In another equine investigation, the results of 100 suspensory injuries that were not treated with bone marrow stem cells were compared the results to 100 horses that had been treated with bone marrow stem cells. In the untreated group, less than 30% went back to work and stayed sound; in the treated group, 80% went back to work and stayed sound for at least one year.

Many injuries treated with stem cell therapy are discrete core lesions of the digital flexor tendons and suspensory ligament. Other applications of stem cell therapy have included check ligament injury, various collateral ligament injuries, cruciate ligament injuries, meniscal injuries of the stifle joint and others. Intra-articular treatment with stem cells has been employed on a more limited basis for conditions such as osteochondrosis dissecans (OCD) cysts involving various joints. Successful therapy with stem cells may be further facilitated with concurrent hyperbaric oxygen therapy. Hyperbaric oxygen therapy has been reported to increase the number of circulating stem cells in blood eightfold. The final goal is not just repair of an injury, but rather, regeneration of normal tissue in damaged areas using stem cell therapy. The current focus of equine stem cell therapy is in tendon and ligamentous injuries. However, there may likely be many other surgical and medical conditions that would benefit from advances in stem cell research and therapy.

A-CELL

The word "A-cell", literally refers to the lack of cells, "acellularity". A-cell is a product that can be described as an extracellular matrix product. Historically, the extracellular matrix has been regarded as primarily inert.. However, the complexity of the extracullular matrix has been more clearly defined and reportedly now includes numerous growth factors, inhibitors and an inherent ability to attract the body's own stem cells to an area of healing for tissue restoration. The A-cell product utilizes this extra cellular matrix milieu and its functional capabilities to provide the scaffolding in the coordination and signaling of tissue repair, regeneration and replacement. The A-Cell Inc. product is derived from pig urinary bladder matrix. Product is prepared by removal of cellular material, leaving only extra-cellular matrix. Bladder tissue was chosen for the production due to the high percentage of extra-cellular matrix relative to cellular material. The A-Cell product takes advantage of these extracellular matrix properties in order to provide the framework and signaling required for homologous circulating stem cells to populate the area of treatment and to differentiate into normal healthy tissue rather than scar tissue. By using this commercial matrix product, one researcher aptly described the introduction of a "mini-ecosystem" into damaged tissue to facilitate tissue healing and regeneration. With further investigation, the A-cell product technology may prove to be universally applicable throughout the body for healing. An initial application of use of the A-cell product was in the form of sheets to facilitate external wound healing. For equine tendon and ligament injuries, the appealing characteristic of A-cell therapy has been promoted as its simplicity for use. A-cell appears to be effective without the need to harvest tissue and isolate stem cells before using them in the horse.

A-cell has been utilized with success for injuries of the suspensory ligament and suspensory branches, superficial and deep flexor tendons, check ligament injuries and other tendons. Following a preliminary diagnosis, the lesion is further evaluated by ultrasonography in order to determine specific location and severity. After resolution of the initial swelling of the injury at 1 week or later, under sedation and surgical prep, the ultrasound is again used to guide direct injection of the reconstituted product directly into the injury site. Therapy with A-cell injection has been reported to produce significant pain following the procedure. This characteristic is believed to occur due to an intense inflammatory response to the procedure. It is presumed that this inflammatory reaction precipitates tissue repair. The expected post-injection response should be clearly outlined with the client. Post-injection pain may be controlled with aggressive anti-inflammatory therapy prior to the procedure. Controlled exercise has also been reported to be helpful to help minimize the amount of swelling occurs after injection. The use of A-cell has been estimated to reduce recovery time by about 30 percent when an appropriate rehabilitation program is in place. Following therapy, the ultrasonographic evaluation of fiber patterns in treated tendons at 60 days have been reported to be similar to the ultrasonographic appearance of fiber patterns seen following stem cell therapy. One researcher involved in the product development reported that the most difficult injuries to treat successfully were those affecting the suspensory branches. The greatest success was reported with proximal suspensory and superficial digital flexor injuries. A-cell is reported to exhibit antibacterial activity. It has been reported to be successfully used to help successfully treat tendon sheath sepsis and to permit the horse to return to athletic use. Because of the frequent encounter of significant local inflammation following its use, therapy with A-cell is utilized judiciously and often with hesitation by some practitioners..

Platelet Rich Plasma (PRP)

Platelet rich plasma (PRP) has been utilized for treatment of equine tendon and ligament injuries. The procedure requires whole blood collection from the horse followed by immediate centrifugation in order to concentrate platelets and circulating growth factors that are believed to improve and speed healing. Many systems are currently available to veterinarians as well as to physicians. Factors such as platelet concentration and purity vary significantly between separation systems. Following resolution of initial swelling, the platelet rich plasma of the centrifuged blood is separated and subsequently injected into a soft tissue lesion using ultrasound guidance. Although PRP appears to provide superior results of healing in comparison to conservative medical management, platelet-rich plasma injection has been reported to lead to more significant scarring of treated ligaments than stem cell bone marrow treatment of comparable lesions. Stem cell enhanced healing appeared to induce healing without causing significant scarring. PRP thereapy is used widely in equine patients at this time.

Hyperbaric Oxygen Therapy (HBOT)

Hyperbaric oxygen therapy (HBOT) is high-dose oxygen inhalation therapy achieved by having the horse breathe 100% oxygen inside a pressurized hyperbaric chamber. Because hyperbaric oxygen is not appreciably absorbed through the skin, tissue oxygen delivery occurs only through normal respiration. Although high tissue-oxygen level is the main therapeutic benefit of HBOT, other reported benefits include reduction of edema, modification of growth factor and cytokine effects, stimulation of capillary budding and granulation tissue formation in the wound bed, promotion of cellular proliferation, acceleration of collagen deposition, and increased microbial oxidative killing. Studies have shown that soft tissue injuries treated with HBOT recover in half the time. Furthermore, increasing oxygen content in ischemic tissue appears to facilitate or even potentiate the activity of antimicrobial agents. HBOT modulates the immune system response and enhances oxygen-radical scavenging to decrease ischemia-reperfusion injury. Hyperbaric oxygenation can be associated with side effects including sensation of pressure in the head, CNS signs and pulmonary irritation. However, preliminary physical examination of the HBOT candidate coupled with the appropriate use of hyperoxia makes this a safest therapeutic intervention.

By far, wounds and bone infections are the most common problems in the horse that are treated with hyperbaric oxygen. The use of hyperbaric oxygen in such cases focuses on an effort to reduce sloughing and loss of tissue. Another area of interest is soft-tissue infections, such as tendon sheath infections. Hyperbaric oxygen treatment in these cases is utilized to enhance antibiotic function and to promote white blood cell destruction of bacteria. Hyperbaric oxygen therapy is considered supportive therapy. Surgical drainage and administration of appropriate antibiotics based on a culture of the infected fluid remain the principal treatments for this type of infection. Acute and chronic conditions salient to the performance horse that are commonly treated with HBOT include; post-surgical and slow healing wounds, tendon and ligament injuries, exercise induced pulmonary hemorrhage, infections, laminitis and navicular syndrome, exertional rhabdomyolysis, nerve trauma and pre and post stem cell surgery patients.

MAGNETIC/ PULSED MAGNETIC THERAPY

Animals and people are electrically charged. All of the cells in the body exhibit a resting electric current known as the cellular electrical potential. The resting electrical potential of a cell is maintained by the cellular membrane. Normal cellular function depends on the cellular membrane's role in maintaining normal cellular potential. By virtue of the numerous charged particles within it, blood is an electrical conductor capable of carrying electric current within the body. When the ions and charged particles pass through a magnetic field, a separation of ions occurs. When a cell suffers traumatic injury, the electrical potential of the cell is believed to increase to about 120 MV or decrease significantly in a cell with a long-standing injury. This is where the efficacy of magnetic therapy comes is believed to work. Among other effects, magnets are believed to cause an increase in blood flow, which is reported to enhance the healing process. The principle that explained the reported effect of magnetic therapy on the blood vessel is called the Hall Effect. This effect states that a potential difference is produced across an electrical conductor, transverse to an electric current in the conductor and a magnetic field perpendicular to the current. The belief of magnetic therapy advocates is that this potential difference is produced in the blood vessel with its current of charges running through it. Static or permanent magnets are proposed to produce three effects on blood vessels. First, there is a slight liberation of heat with ionic separation. Second, the ions cross back and forth between the North and South poles of the magnet. Third, small eddy currents are produced in the bloodstream. These effects, collectively contribute to widening of the blood vessels, which allows more blood to pass through. At the same time, thermal energy is produced that contributes to an increase in regional blood flow, oxygenation, and supply of nutrients. A reduction in the production of toxic metabolic byproducts with their concurrently improved removal occurs with better perfusion. Heat generation is reported to help modulate pain through the vascular changes and through proposed neurological changes. This neurological control of pain is explained by "gate control theory". Pain signals are believed to be blocked if the sensory afferent neurons are sufficiently stimulated. The application of heat, or other stimulation, to an injured part might sufficiently overload the pain transmission with a preponderance of sensory input from thermoreceptors. It has also been noted that vascular changes reduce pain by accelerating the natural heating process. Heat production itself also contributes to vasodilation. A supportive laboratory investigation into the vascular effects of magnetic therapy suggested that magnetic therapy could significantly bebefit circulatory flow. The mediators responsible for propagation of the pain-spasm-pain cycle are also removed from the area by increased blood flow. The pain modulation effect of magnetic therapy has been supported by an equine study that suggested an analgesic effect of magnetic therapy as measured by hoof withdrawl pain reflex.

There are two common types of magnetic therapy. Both forms of treatment are non-invasive and essentially pain-free. Although proponents agree that both forms of therapy are beneficial, there is disagreement to which form of therapy is superior. The first type is administered with a common static or permanent magnet. The magnetic field in a static magnet does not change. Static magnets used in human magnetic therapy normally fall between 300 and 500 Gauss. Magnetic resonance imaging (MRI), used in medicine to view structures inside the body, introduces a strong magnetic field in excess of 10,000 Gauss. Because the magnetic fields acting on the blood vessels are required to be oriented perpendicular to the vessels, the available magnetic pole patterns were inefficient because they failed to recognize anatomic variations. Blood vessels do not travel in straight or predictable paths. One's blood vessels comprise a meshwork, running in several different directions within any given area. The available patterns were either a series of alternate poles arranged on a parallel design, or they were magnetized with one pole covering an entire surface or its opposite surface was oppositely magnetized. A design of a series of concentric circles of alternate magnetic poles represents the most efficient pattern conceivable. This pattern ensures that other than vessels running perpendicular to the skin, every blood vessel will cross a series of North-South poles. The second form of magnetic therapy is administered with an electromagnet. Electromagnetic or pulsed magnetic therapy is provided by the use of padded magnetic coils that are attached to a source of electricity such as a battery or an outlet. The patient side of the coil has a magnetic south pole polarity during the first half cycle of the ringing magnetic field pulse. Treatment of a horse requires placement of the coil over the area of concern for anywhere from 5 to 15 minutes. The frequency of pulsations delivered using pulsed electromagnetic devices is measured in cycles per second (Hertz). The strength of the magnet is measured in Gauss. Pulsating magnetic therapy can be controlled by the therapist as to frequency of pulsations (Hertz), the intensity of the pulse (Gauss), and the duration of treatment. Because of the ability to control these 3 variables, pulsed electromagnetic devices are becoming popular in equine sports medicine. Healing is believed to be accelerated by simulating normal tissue resonance in both Gauss units and the frequency in Hertz. As in laser therapy, the frequency used depends on the type of injury. In general, low frequency settings are used on acute injury, medium frequencies are used to balance and restore energy, and high frequencies are used on old, cold injuries and scars. As mentioned, it is theorized that magnetic therapy can relieve pain by stimulating nerve fibers, which, in essence, shut down pain transmission. Pulsed magnetic therapy has been proposed to produce several beneficial effects in living tissue. These effects are; charge density waves, electrical eddy currents, lymph fluid movement by involuntary muscle contraction, and the conversion of fibroblast cells of scar tissue, or that are to become scar tissue, into embryonic-type cells that reportedly can convert into normal healthy tissue (referred to as "dedifferentiation of fibroblast cells"). Tissue or scar tissue is thereby believed to be repaired/removed and to be replaced with normal healthy tissue. The charge density waves and induction of electrical eddy currents in intracellular fluids are also reported to exhibit antimicrobial (bacteria and viruses) activity when they enter the range of 100 microamperes per square centimeter to 200,000 microamperes per square centimeter. Antimicrobial effect is believed to be produced by virtue of the effect of the charge density wave disruption of the configuration of proteins on the surface of bacteria and viruses, rendering ineffective the attachment and receptor proteins of the microbes. Through this process of protein denaturation, the effects of the pulsed magnetic therapy are also believed to inactivate toxins. Lymph flow is reported to be facilitated by electric field induction of motor axon fibers and the resultant induction of involuntary muscular contraction. The muscle contraction perpetuates the lymph movement through the vessels that run through and around muscle tissue.

Pulsed magnetic fields are proposed to offer diagnostic utility in addition to the therapeutic effects already outlined. Because collagenous scar tissue is believed to exhibit significant ability to conduct electrical current, exposure of collagen rich scar tissue to the pulsed magnetic field of the coil, electric currents are induced in and throughout the scar tissue. It is believed that sensory nerve fibers in this region are stimulated and the horse experiences a stabbing sensation at the site of tissue damage each time the coil rings. Slowly moving the coil over the entire horse's body surface most tissue damaged regions or areas can be located. Poorly innervated tissue and areas of the body with no tissue damage but where the horse still senses the coil pulse (face, head and sacral areas) are situations where the diagnostic potential of the pulsed magnet would not be expected to be useful. Horses must be acclimated to the use and sensation of the pulsed magnet. If the sensation of the pulse is too intense for the horse to apparently tolerate, an increase in the distance from the coil to the tissue may help alleviate the perceived intensity. This can be achieved by the placement of a pillow or a blanket between the coil and the patient, or by just holding the coil further from the animal.

People with pacemakers, or cochlear hearing implants cannot use or be near a pulsed magnet fear of damaging the device. Furthermore, all cell phones, land line phones, TV remotes, watches, and anything that might be damaged by an intense high voltage surge must be kept at least ten feet away from the coil when such a magnet is in use. Any item capable of conducting electricity in a closed path, such as chains and necklaces, cannot be worn for fear of sparking between links (in poorly conductive regions). Caution must also be taken when treating horses in or around stalls constructed with metal. The pulsed magnetic field will induce eddy currents in that closed electrical pathway each time the pulsed magnet is fired. The magnetic field expands and contracts through the closed electrical path way each time the pulsed magnet is fired. If the closed electrical path has a poorly conductive region such as a cracked and/or rusted weld, then a large shower of sparks can be generated at this site of the defective electrical conduction.

Physiotherapeutic Modalities

The objective of physiotherapy is to increase the possibility of tissue repair by using the properties of heat, ultrasound waves, electricity, and cold, in order to stimulate natural physiological processes. Conditions that are believed to benefit from physiotherapy may include; muscular spasm or tightness, muscle strain, muscle weakness, spinal pain or stiffness, soft tissue injuries, nerve injuries, wound healing, some orthopedic conditions, training and performance problems, compensatory conditions, behavioral changes, saddle problems and post-surgical rehabilitation. Some techniques utilized in physiotherapy include; soft tissue mobilisation, manipulation, massage, range of motion stretching, pain relief modalities, muscle stimulation, exercise therapy, muscle and gait re-education, laser therapy, ultrasound, H-Wave, TENS, and magnetic field therapy. Some of the more commonly utilized modes of physiotherapy have been covered in separate sections in this chapter. These techniques of treating injuries of soft tissue or bone structures have been, and are still, widely used in human athletes. Although some protocols have been used in the treatment of injuries in the sport horse, there is at the present time, minimal scientific data to directly support specific physiotherapeutic modalities in horses.

Electrotherapy using Transcutaneous Electrical Nerve Stimulators (TENS), is a modality of physiotherapy utilized to help modulate pain. Tens machines transmit an electrical current through a patient's affected areas. The electrical current is transmitted through electrodes that are placed on the skin. The central idea behind electrotherapy is that by interfering with pain signaling, analgesia can be induced. TENS machines allow you to adjust the amount of current to find the optimal levels for each patient. Depending on the frequency of the pulse, it is also possible to use electrical current to trigger endorphins, thereby providing additional pain relief. The current produces a tingling sensation that in turn influences pain pathways. The spinal cord is part of the central nervous system and together with the sensory nerves, it sends pain signals to the brain. Ideally, the electrical current will block pain receptors in the brain, and the patient will feel his or her pain lessening, often after half an hour. Tens Machines are reported to be effective for the relief of pain, and are a great alternative to medical therapy. TENS therapy is also reported to be useful for muscle development, deep tissue release, breaking down adhesions and scarring and helping the horse relax.

H-wave therapy is applied using a specific instrument for electrotherapeutic treatment in pain control and functional restoration. H-Wave ultra low frequency protocols are based on the principle that fluid shifts and pressures are essential for tissues healing and homeostasis. The H-Wave device was specifically designed to improve circulation and enhance fluid shifts in order to address inflammation as the causative factor in pain. The H-Wave machine creates comfortable and strong muscle contractions. A 30 minute treatment will contract muscles and is believed to increase fluid shifts in the treatment area. H-Wave therapy is not designed to mask symptoms while the equipment is on, but rather to speed recovery and/or manage chronic symptoms by instituting several 30 minute treatments per day/week, as prescribed. Some conditions may require additional pain relief that fluid shifts due with ultra low frequency stimulation do not produce. The commercially available H-Wave instrument is equipped with a second, high frequency mode that focuses on shutting down pain and breaking the pain cycle. This setting is not intended to mask pain while the device is on, but rather to create an anesthetic affect with significant, lasting relief beyond the 30 minute treatment. Reportedly, unlike a TENS machine, H-Wave is reported to be rehabilitative and to produce long lasting pain relief and benefit from a 30 minute treatment.

Therapeutic ultrasound is another form of physiotherapy used to produce microvibration and deep heating of tissue to facilitate blood flow, fibroblast stimulation, absorption of edema, relieve pain, accelerate tissue repair and modify scar formation. Clinical applications of ultrasound therapy include soft tissue injury from acute conditions such as sports injuries, ligament sprains, tendonitis, subacute conditions such as bursitis and capsulitis, chronic conditions including osteoarthritis, wounds, ulcers such as pressure sores, and treatment and control of pain such as back pain. These conditions fall into three broad groups of physiotherapy; musculoskeletal/orthopaedic physiotherapy (which includes manipulative physiotherapy and sports/exercise physiotherapy), respiratory and neurologic physiotherapy. As with most forms of physiotherapy, anecdotal reports of success are poorly substantiated by research that demonstrates clearly beneficial effects of the modality.

Laser therapy is a form of physiotherapy produced by cellular exposure to laser energy in order to induce changes in cellular homeostasis. The laser energy is proposed to induce a cascade of reactions that influence several components of the respiratory chain including cytochromes and cytchrome oxidase. These molecules are the primary laser acceptors capable of absorbing the therapeutic wavelengths. A short term activation of the respiratory chain presumably leads to changes in redox status and enhanced synthesis of ATP. The laser energy absorption is believed to affect hydrogen ion levels in the cell and in combination with increased ATP, affects cell permeability and ionic flow of sodium, potassium, and calcium. These changes are deemd to be necessary to control the proliferative activity of the cell. The induced healing effects of laser therapy are reported to include increased cell metabolism, improved local blood circulation, development of collagen and muscle tissue, relief of both acute and chronic pain, reduction in local inflammation and edema, stimulation of wound healing and tissue repair, stimulation of the immune system and promotion of nerve function.

The benefits of methodically increasing range of motion in the prevention of muscle and tendon pulls are well recognized in human sports medicine. However, this practice has long been overlooked in equine athletic performance. Providing a horse with a stretch routine may help to significantly increase the range of motion of muscle groups. The resultant tissue elasticity may significantly reduce the chances of injury and improve performance. Incorrect stretching can either injure your horse or impede optimal performance. However, any owner or trainer can learn the basics of stretching and serve the role of the physiotherapist for manual stretching exercises. The front legs are stretched by picking up, the leg and gently flexing at the ankle three or four times. Then, the knee is flexed by bending the entire lower leg up and down while keeping the ankle and knee parallel to the elbow. Next the foreleg is pulled forward and down while standing in front of the horse and supporting the leg from below the ankle. Subsequently, the lower limb is folded the lower leg back up towards the elbow while the therapist moves to the horse's side, followed by extension of the lower leg down while applying pressure to the dorsum of the knee to stretch the leg back and down towards the hind foot. The hind legs are stretched by first flexing the ankle as performed in the foreleg. Follow this maneuver with stretching of the hind limb forward and downward while directing the hind foot towards the heel of the front foot. The therapist then moves to the back of the horse facing the hindlimbs. While the foot in hand, the leg is slowly stretched caudally with a free hand in place on the back of the hock in a very strict straight caudal motion. The remaining hindlimb stretch is performed from the opposite side of the horse. The hindlimb being stretched is lifted by the foot and gently pulled towards the heel of the front foot on the same side as the therapist. In order to stretch the back muscles, the therapist starts caudally by flexing the tail from its base so the horse relaxes his tail and back. Tail clamping or resistance to flexion may indicate a sore back or other related problem affecting the back. The therapist then gently and gradually pulls outward using a grasp of the tail near the tip of the tail bone. The strength of the pull is gradually increased and the horse is encouraged to lean forward against the pull. The pull strength is slowly and gradually released in order to prevent sudden release. Bending of the axial skeleton is also a beneficial stretching exercise.

It may be helpful to have the horse stand against a wall in order to help prevent excess movement during the therapy. With the therapist standing next to the horse at a point near the elbow, the neck is either gently flexed towards the elbow, or an enticement is provided for him to voluntarily flex to the point of the elbow. Reluctance and/or resistance to this maneuver may indicate axial or upper appendicular discomfort. Rounding the back is a stretch of the epaxial muscles induced by pressing into the abdomen in the area of the umbilicus to induce movement away from the stimulus by rounding the back. A final stretch focuses on the flexion and rounding of the neck downwards in order to stretch the dorsal neck muscles. This stretch is only performed by the horse voluntarily and therefore requires an enticement such as a carrot, grain or green grass or hay. The enticement is shown to the horse in hand and is used to lead the horse's head to reach between and through the forelegs.

Massage is arguably the most natural means of helping to alleviate pain. Throughout history, many systems and theories concerning the management of musculoskeletal pain and dysfunction have come and gone, but employment of massage therapy has remained. They styles of Swedish massage and sports massage each includes the techniques of effleurage, kneading or petrissage, and percussion. The techniques are applied in specific order in order to impact the circulatory, respiratory, muscular and nervous systems. Massage therapy may be utilized in a variety of applications. A maintenance performance massage can be a combination of swedish massage and sports massage techniques. The focus of maintenance performance massage is to produce effects leading to stress reduction, relaxation and performance enhancement. The result is believed to be increased circulation to the muscles and tendons facilitating suppleness and quieting of the nervous system. Applying performance maintenance massage weekly, bi-weekly or monthly, may help prevent repetitive use injuries, enhance endurance and maintain flexibility. Maintenance performance massage is recommended no sooner than three days prior to performance in order to permit adjustment to body changes that occur during and after the massage. Pre-event and post-even massage therapies are each tailored for distinct purposes. These massage styles are to be applied on the day of competition or strenuous workout. Pre-event massage is utilized in order to enhance warm-up, not substitute it. The theoretical benefit of pre-event massage is to fill the muscles with well-oxygenated, nutrient filled blood by increasing circulation. The result is thought to be improvement in tissue suppleness and metabolic exchange and reduced muscle and mental tension. Kneading techniques such as deep compressions, and cross fibering techniques are often heavily utilized for pre-event massage. Deep compressions may also be performed to further facilitate circulation to the muscles. Post-event massage focuses on helping to reduce the effects of muscular trauma sustained during competition and workouts. The reported objective is to purge toxins released from heavy muscle activity. It is believed that this helps tissue recover more quickly and facilitates continued performance. Cross fiber frictions are used to release adhesions or scar tissue believed to result from small micro-tears in muscle. The other techniques commonly employed in post-event massage include effleurage and deep compression. Effleurage is employed by long stroking movements that facilitate movement of blood through the veins. It is promoted to help flush the toxins from the muscles by increasing circulation to the area. Deep compressions are used in conjunction with effleurage in order to promote the removal of waste products.

One of the least controversial modalities of physiotherapy is probably the use of cold therapy. The reason for the acceptance of cold therapy is its widely accepted physiological effects that include; peripheral vasoconstriction followed by vasodilatation of the deep tissues, analgesia, reduction in muscular spasm, reduced tissue enzymatic activity and a decrease in edema and inflammation. The advantages of cold therapy in sport horse tendon injuries have long been recognized and utilized. However, the methods of application and efficacy of cold therapy are as numerous as they are varied. The simplest procedures are cold water hosing, or application of ice packs. Other methods include cooling boots with circulating water, commercial bandages or leg wraps made of material which maintains a low temperature after withdrawal from the freezer, refrigerated leg garters and others. The recommended duration of application of this therapy appears to vary with the product or device utilized.. These recommendations include applications anywhere from 10 minutes up to 60 minutes. Some studies have been conducted to analyze the various methods of cold application. The conclusions of some studies suggested that certain methods failed to maintain the cold temperature for long enough duration, the cold temperature around the site of inflammation would rapidly rise and limit the therapeutic effect of cold therapy.

Cryotherapy has been proposed as a more effective method of providing the benefit of cold therapy to horses with various sports related injuries. Gas cryotherapy has been proposed as potentially useful for the utilization of cryotherpeutics. The benefits of cryotherapy beyond cold therapy are reported to include a sharp and immediate interruption of acute inflammation, significant analgesia, significant reduction in edema, rapid regression of hematic infiltrates, rapid increase in blood flow in the area of the tendon and improved quality of scar repair tissue. This mode of treatment has been utilized in a very limited basis to treat horses diagnosed with superficial digital flexor tendon injuries, suspensory injuries, muscle trauma, supra-spinous ligament injury and chronic joint disease. Further investigation into the application of cryotherapy is necessary to make any conclusions. It is possible that this mode of therapy could prove to be helpful, particularly if used as an emergency intervention to immediately help control the damage to structures injured in athletic performance.

Specific Homeopathic Therapies (Zeel, Traumeel, Injeel)

Produced in Germany, Zeel-T (Heel, Inc.) contains 15 homeopathic medicines in a diluted form consistent with standard homeopathic principles. In horses and humans, Zeel is primarily used to manage joint pain and inflammation. The individual ingredients are formulated to work synergistically to show distinct inhibitory effects on the production of LTB4 by 5-lipoxygenase and on the synthesis of PGE-2 by COX-1 and COX-2 enzymes. Zeel is available in ointment, tablet, oral vial and prescription injectable formulations. Several authors have demonstrated dual inhibition of 5-lipoxygenase/cyclooxygenase. Research articles have also noted its favorable gastrointestinal tolerability over the use of traditional NSAIDs. Overall, studies have shown the product is safe and as effective as Cox-1 and Cox-2 inhibitors. A comparison of Zeel combination homeopathic injection to NSAIDs in the reduction of joint pain in patients with degenerative joint disease found uniform improvement in patient symptoms with both treatments. Injectable Zeel has been mixed with either bupivacaine (Marcaine) or lidocaine for the treatment of degenerative joint disease in the first metatarsophalangeal joint, subtalar arthritis and other degenerative joint disease pathology of the lower extremity in humans. It has also been reported to work well for psoriatic arthritis and rheumatoid arthritis. Zeel has been used in humans for both periarticular and intraarticular injection. Zeel injectable is isotonic in nature and produces minimal pain with injection even without an anesthetic. In humans with first MPJ degenerative changes and chronic pain, intraarticular injection of 1 cc of the Zeel medication has been used to control clinical signs. With acute pain in the joint, a periarticular injection of the medication mixed with a local anesthetic is performed. There is no precipitation or flocculation that occurs when mixing Zeel-T with lidocaine or bupivacaine. In human patients, these injections can be administered weekly without any danger of adverse reactions or soft tissue instability that may be seen with steroid injections. Continue therapy can be prescribed by oral therapy using the same homeopathic medicine (Zeel oral tablets) and/or the topical cream (Zeel ointment), that have similar homeopathic constituents to the injectable form. Zeel can be administered to a patient concomitantly with NSAIDs without any additive adverse effects including those of the gastrointestinal or cardiovascular or renal systems. At least one human study demonstrated that combined allopathic and homeopathic treatment utilizing Zeel-T and diclofenac produced greater and longer lasting improvement in symptoms. It was noted in the same study that the combination of these modalities proved especially effective in treating periarthritis and mild to moderate synovitis in human patients with advanced osteoarthritis of the knee.

Traumeel is another homeopathic product produced by Heel Inc. Traumeel is available as a topical ointment, as oral tablets, oral drops, oral liquid in vials, and as an injectable (prescription only). Traumeel is used in horses and humans for soft tissue inflammation and pain. The mechanism of action of Traumeel Injection Solution appears to be the result of modulation of the release of oxygen radicals from activated neutrophils, and the inhibition of the release of inflammatory mediators (possibly interleukin-1 from activated macrophages) and neuropeptides. Therefore, Traumeel is an anti-inflammatory, analgesic, anti-edematous, anti-exudative combination of 12 botanical and 2 mineral substances. Traumeel is indicated for the temporary relief of symptoms associated with inflammatory, exudative, and degenerative processes due to acute trauma including; contusions, lacerations, fractures, sprains, post-operative wounds, repetitive or overuse injuries including tendinitis, bursitis, epicondylitis, and for the temporary relief of minor aches and pains associated with such conditions. Traumeel is also indicated for the temporary relief of minor aches and pains associated with backache, muscular aches, and the minor pain from rheumatoid arthritis, osteoarthritis, gouty arthritis, and ankylosing spondylitis. The clinical efficacy of Traumeel is supported by scientific research and years of worldwide usage. For example, a randomized, double-blind, placebo-controlled study of Traumeel Ointment for the treatment of ankle sprains found that patients treated with Traumeel were pain free and had a greater range of motion sooner than the control group. Of 107 homeopathic studies reviewed by Kleijnen et al., the Zell study of Traumeel ranked within the top 5% for methodological quality. A meta-analysis of homeopathic studies in another respected medical journal reported three different controlled studies that demonstrated the effectiveness of Traumeel over placebo. The homeopathic contents of Traumeel include the following ingredients paired with their activities:

- Neurogenic phase–Aconitum –paraesthesia, neuralgia, formication (An abnormal sensation as of needling or light pricking in or upon the skin; a common symptom in diseases of the spinal cord and the peripheral nerves); Hypericum -Nerve-like sensation -pain in area where there are lots of nerves

- Vascular phase –Arnica -Sore, bruised pain; Hamamelis –severe soreness, vein issues (hemorrhage, bruising); Belladonna -Throbbing pain –rapid onset
- Exudation –Bellis –Hemorrhage, hematoma
- Neutrophil Migration –Mercuriussolubilis–for highly acute inflammation; Hepar sulphuris–tendency toward abscesses
- Lymphocyte Migration–Echinacea –inflammation of every kind & feverish infections
- Resorption & Reconstruction –Calendula –cuts, jagged, torn; puffy & oozing; Symphytum-non-union fractures & blunt trauma

CONCLUSION

Non-articular therapies include any and all techniques directed at controlling or treating lameness, but that do not require intra-articular injection. Non-articular therapies may include wellresearched and proven modes of therapy. However, less well understood and proven treatment modalities are also commonly employed. Such therapeutic approaches have greatly expanded over the last several years. For the equine practitioner, it is easy to be skeptical about the therapeutic benefit of the myriad of these therapies that are now available. This is because, for many of these treatments, there is minimal or no clinical research or objective report regarding their efficacy. However, today's practitioner, especially the performance horse practitioner, must work with many individuals who not only believe in these therapies, but also actively advocate and market them. An open mind is required to successfully and helpfully integrate and to provide advice on non-articular and "alternative" therapies. As a result, many equine practitioners have developed significant confidence in the use of some of these therapies. Overall, recommendations for non-articular therapy may include a mixture of recognized, researched and proven treatment techniques in addition to poorly understood and proven modalities of therapy. The utilization of such treatments is generally guided by the preferences and experiences of the veterinarian and owner.

REFERENCES

[1] Bryant J, Milne R. *Therapeutic ultrasound in physiotherapy*. Bristol: NHS Executive South and West; 1998 December. Development and Evaluation Committee Report No.: 90: 1-21.

[2] Caron JP. *Large Animal Veterinary Rounds:* Therapy for Equine Joint Disease. 2006. Available from: www.canadianveterinarians.net /larounds.

[3] Carter J, Carter GK, Easter JL, Frisbie D, McClure S, Mitchell RD. *Managing equine joint inflammation: A roundtable discussion on diagnostic and treatment options*. Suppl Compend Cont Ed Pract Vet; Equine Edition 2(3)A; 2007; 1-16.

[4] CEVA *Sante Animale.* Tildren. 2003. Available from: http://www.tildren.com/tildrenhome.nsf

[5] CEVA *Sante Animale.* Tildren 500 mg Infusion. Marketing brochure; Animal Health LTD, Chesham, Bucks; 2008; 1-10.

[6] Chay S, Woods WE, Nugent TE, Weckman T, Sprinkle F, Blake JW, Tobin T, Soma LR,Yocum J, et al. Population distributions of phenylbutazone and oxyphenbutazone after oral and i.v. doing in horses. *J Vet Pharmacol Ther*; 1984; 7(4): 265-276.
[7] Dowling PM. *Myths and truths about controlling pain and inflammation in horses.* Available from:www.distanceriding.org/php/articles/health/ Inflammation; 1-10.
[8] Gerring EL, Lees P, Taylor JB. Pharmacokinetics of phenylbutazone and its metabolites in the horse. *Equine Vet J*; 1981; 13(3):152-157.
[9] Herbots P. *Physiotherapy.* In: 21de Studiedag van de / 21ème Journée d'étude de la Belgian Equine Practitioners Society. Liege, Belgium; 2004; 1-5.
[10] Herthel DJ. *Enhanced suspensory ligament healing in100 horses by stem cells and other bone marrow components:* Proceedings of the 47th annual convention of the American Association of Equine Practitioners; 2001.
[11] Haussler KK. Equine *Chiropractic: General Principles and Clinical Applications.* In Proceed 46th Meeting Amer Assoc Equine Pract; 2000; 84-93.
[12] Keegan KG, Messer NT, Reed SK, Wilson DA, Kramer J. Effectiveness of administration of phenylbutazone alone or concurrent administration of phenylbutazone and flunixin meglumine to alleviate lameness in horses. *AJVR*; 2008; 69(2): 167-173.
[13] Rabine JP. *Benefits of treating sport horse locomotor apparatus lesions with cryonic medical advanced cryotherapy: A new therapeutic technology in equine physiotherapy.* Avaiable from: www.mtavet.com/cryo/downloads/EquineWhitePaper.pdf: Cryonic Medical, Inc., Montecito, CA.; 1-27.
[14] Rozen D, Parvez U. *Pulsed radiofrequency of lumbar nerve roots for treatment of chronic inguinal herniorraphy pain.* Pain Physician; 2006 Apr;9(2):153-6.
[15] Tobin T, Chay S, Kamerling S, Woods WE, Weckman TJ, Blake JW, Lees P. Pheyylbutazone in the horse: a review. *J Vet Pharmacol Ther*; 1986; 9(1):1-25.
[16] Tóth F, Schumacher J, Schramme M, Kelly G. Proximal Suspensory Desmitis of the Hindlimbs. *Compendium Equine* 4(7); 2009; 308-318.
[17] *United States Equestrian Federation.* Drugs and Medication Guidelines. 2007: 1-29.
[18] Unknown. *Corticosteroid- Glucocorticoid Effects (Veterinary—Systemic);* The United States Pharmacopeial Convention; 2004; 1-67.

In: Rehabilitating the Athletic Horse
Editors: H. W. Jann et al., pp. 159-177
ISBN: 978-1-678-1-60876-672-7

Chapter 8

CONTROLLED EXERCISE STRATEGIES

Hank Jann[1], Rob Glass[2] and Suzanne M. Konz[3]

[1]DVM, MS, Diplomate ACVS, Equine Surgery. College of Veterinary Medicine. Oklahoma State University, Oklahoma, USA

[2]MSCC, Strength and Conditioning Coach, Oklahoma State University, Oklahoma, USA

[3]ATC, CSCS, PhD, Kinesiologist, Colvin Recreation Center, Stillwater, Oklahoma, USA

ABSTRACT

Although no conditioning strategy can be universally applied to all horses, there are some fundamental principles that should be followed when devising a conditioning strategy for a given individual. This chapter highlights the major concepts involved in conditioning a horse for competition and for reconditioning a horse during rehabilitation. The major focus is on developing a foundation and then adding to this with more intensified and specialized advanced forms of conditioning to develop strength, speed, stamina, and plyometrics. The concepts contained in this chapter can be applied to all equine disciplines.

INTRODUCTION

Controlled exercise forms the basis of preparation for athletic competition, and for rehabilitating the injured athlete. This chapter describes the fundamental components of athletic conditioning and of reconditioning following injury. We have included basic conditioning strategies at the beginning of the chapter because fundamental knowledge of athletic conditioning is required before rehabilitation strategies can be devised. The underlying premise of this chapter is that the incidence of athletic injury is directly related to fatigue, and that the latter devolves from insufficient or ineffective physical conditioning. In fact, the most powerful tool available in the prevention of athletic injury is adequate conditioning prior to competition. Our ability to rehabilitate an injured athlete is directly related to the expertise utilized in designing and implementing conditioning strategies. This chapter will provide conditioning strategies for athletic horses. It will also provide conditioning programs for humans not only by way of comparison, but also because the equine trainer can benefit from adapting these strategies to horses.

Strategy for Basic Conditioning

Foundation

The term foundation refers to a concept that should pervade all conditioning strategies regardless of the athletic endeavor. In the simplest of possible terms, it constitutes "getting in shape so you can get in shape." Foundation is the *sine qua non* of all successful conditioning strategies. Lack thereof effectively dooms any such plan to failure. Of all the errors we make in conditioning, the lack of building a firm foundation is the most grievous, because it impacts upon all future progress. Sadly, foundation is also the component of a conditioning strategy that is the most often neglected because it is time-consuming and expensive. The general concept of foundation actually varies very little between athletic disciplines. The goal is to get the musculoskeletal, cardiovascular, nervous, and heat regulatory systems upgraded to adapt to a regimen of more advanced conditioning. The athlete with an appropriate foundation will not suffer physical and mental exhaustion with its associated sore muscles, joints, and bones as he/she progresses to more advanced training. These ailments typically plague individuals that advance too rapidly into a conditioning program – they lack foundation. A conditioning program that produces the hallmark signs of too rapid advancement, i.e. sore muscles, sore joints or bones, and mental dullness, is one that will in all likelihood fail due to injury. An athlete should be able to advance through the various stages of training smoothly and without setback. Failure to achieve this represents a training error that has a high probability of producing injury. This is true regardless of discipline for animal or human being. Although it might, at first, seem logical to outline different foundation strategies for different individuals (disciplines), this actually is not necessary. A simple foundation outline is adequate. The genetic potential of any given individual will affect the rate of progression through his/ her foundation strategy. Some athletes will adapt rapidly and others will not. In fact, it is in this initial stage of training that the individuals that will be able to perform are identified, and athletic training is either modified or discontinued. Not all individuals have the mental and physical genetic makeup to perform athletically. This is true for both human beings and animals. An astute trainer will recognize this in the early stages of conditioning. Individuals that successfully acquire this introductory foundation can progress toward a more specialized form of training, appropriate to their chosen discipline.

The following is a conditioning program that will achieve foundation in horses. It is meant to serve as a guide and not an inflexible gospel. This strategy can be modified to fit all young-adult and adult horses, regardless of breed. In a perfect world, it would be the routine with which a young horse was started. It is a 12-week strategy, which, if completed, will result in a horse that is ready to initiate more advanced specialized training. Note: In horses, as in humans, there are countless mental issues that must be addressed in order to achieve the desired level of fitness. Often a skilled horseman can train through these issues much the way a skilled coach can counsel a tentative human athlete through various situations encountered in practice or competition. Throughout this book we stress that it can be mental rather than physical issues that slow progress in any conditioning strategy.

Level One

Week 1 Goal: Make Friends with your Horse

A trainer (handler) must determine the kind of animal he has in his care and establish a relationship with it. The quality of that relationship depends on the skill and insight of the trainer. The horse should look to the trainer (handler) as a confident leader (partner) and not as a nervous boss or impatient bully. Notc: not everyone can establish a relationship with an individual horse or any horse and not everyone can be a successful trainer. A good trainer knows (through instinct, experience or both) how hard to push a horse and will do things to build confidence at each stage of the conditioning strategy. It is during this time that things like foot handling, saddle fitting, beginning to lunge, trailer loading and hauling, and establishing familiarity and confidence in the conditioning area are perfected. A horse that is frightened by certain objects in the environment (e.g. cars, busses, bicycles, hay bales, tractors, balloons, flags, loud music, billboards, oil wells, gun fire, exuberant crowds, or other animals) should be slowly but surely desensitized to them. In addition, familiarity with obstacles (conditions) like water, bridges, gates, mud, snow, ice, other horses, and other people should be part of foundation conditioning.[1]

Week 2 Goal: Start Controlled Exercise and Continue to Build Confidence

An appropriate exercise rider is selected – this individual must be dedicated to the task and committed to the individual animal. It is desirable to select light (165 pounds maximum) individuals of medium or below average height. Tall riders can cause fatigue by creating unnatural biomechanical forces due to leverage that the horse must overcome. Exercise riders should be experienced horsemen or horsewomen. It is also desirable that they have an athletic background. They may come from a variety of different disciplines (e.g. race track, endurance, western performance or rodeo, or equitation), but they must have one thing in common: the ability to withstand long periods of mounted training without becoming fatigued themselves. A tired rider will not move with the horse and can become “dead weight” on the horse’s back. This situation leads to undue fatigue of the horse and possible injury. Equally important is that the fatigued rider might make errors in judgment that could jeopardize the welfare of the horse and the entire conditioning strategy. A horse will only get as fit as the exercise rider unless multiple riders are employed and this is logistically difficult in most equine venues other than the racetrack.

Riding exercise is begun using two gaits – the halt and the walk. The mere act of accepting the weight of the rider is a physical effort for the horse that is too often overlooked. It is similar to a weightlifter gaining balance under the bar before attempting a lift or a farrier getting the appropriate balance and grip on an anvil before attempting to carry it. Multiple repetitions of controlled mounting and dismounting strengthen the epaxial and hypaxial

---

[1] Note: It may be that none of these issues can be mastered in the first week. In fact, it may take several weeks or months to reach that point. The trainer must remain aware of the mental issues existent within any given horse, and constantly try to overcome them throughout the entire foundation period.

muscles as well as the sacroiliac ligamentous structures. During and after mounting, the horse should not be allowed to walk off voluntarily until it is cued by the rider. This allows all musculoskeletal effort to begin in a controlled manner – similar to a running back coming out of a three point stance or a sprinter coming out of the starting blocks. These principles are just as important, or even more so, when injured horses are put back in work.

Walking exercise is measured in distance, not time. All exercise distances should be timed and recorded – even if it is as simple as determining how many laps around an arena constitutes a mile. It is a well-recognized fact that an experienced rider carries a clock in his/her head but it is still advisable to time and record all distances. The actual distance an unfit horse walks on the first day should not exceed 2 miles. It should be performed in a controlled manner (steady even pace with a relaxed and confident horse) over flat, even ground. An arena or training track is ideal but an open field or dirt (not gravel) road can provide an excellent training atmosphere as well. The ideal surface over which to begin exercise is dirt, grass, or well-packed sand. These surfaces will avoid foot soreness and possible bruising. Trails may not be ideal due to rocky or uneven surfaces or breaks in terrain that an unfit horse might have difficulty negotiating.

All exercise under tack should be performed on an alternate day basis. This means that, following a day of ridden exercise the horse is given a "day off". The "day off" is just as important to the overall strategy as the conditioning day. This is time to work on overcoming any mental issues that have been recognized during the previous day of training. It also provides rest to allow muscles to recover from fatigue and soreness. Walking exercise should be continued on an alternate day basis for the remainder of the week.

Week 3 Goal: Continue to Walk, Add Distance, Work on Confidence, and Keep the Horse Happy with New Routine

Walking exercise is continued. Times and distances are recorded. The time should show that the speed did not change only the distance. The horse is walking the same speed for an additional mile if his original distance was 2 miles. The horse is now walking 3 miles every other day. The "off days" are still used to address mental issues that may have been recognized and remain unresolved and to allow the horse to recover from the previous day's workout.

Level 2

Week 4 Goal: Continue to Walk, Add Distance, Add Jogging or Trotting to the Routine, Build Confidence and Keep the Horse Happy

Walking exercise is continued at the same speed but another mile is added so the horse is now walking 4 miles every other day. Jogging is added at this time also. The slow jog is performed in a controlled manner for a mile in the middle of the exercise session. The overall work would be walk 2 miles, jog a mile, and then walk 2 more miles. Note: because the exercise sessions have become longer it might be advisable to work in the company of another horse. Most horses seem more confident when they train with other horses. This can serve as a training aid as the distances traveled gradually lengthen.

Week 5 Goal: Keep Walking Distance the Same but Double Jogging Distance, Work on Confidence and Keep the Horse Happy

The horse should now be able to walk 2 miles, jog 2 miles, and walk 2 miles. The walking is intended to increase muscular strength. Increasing jogging distances stresses the cardiovascular, respiratory, and thermoregulatory systems. The nervous system is also stressed because the horse has to learn to jog for an extended period without "breaking gait" i.e. slowing down due to fatigue or "running off" due to lack of confidence. As before, this work is performed on alternate days. It is imperative to continue to work on confidence, since as horses begin to gain fitness they usually become more reactive to external stimuli. Also, trainers need to pay attention to surroundings. A stimulus that did not cause a flight reaction at the walk can produce this at the jog.

Weeks 6-8 Goal: Introduce Hill Work, Increase Jogging Distance on a Weekly Basis, Vary Training Locations if Possible, and Work on Confidence

At this stage of conditioning, the objective is to increase strength by adding hills to the initial 2 mile walking phase of the workout. Jogging is also increased one mile/week. By the end of this phase, the horse will do 2 miles of hill work, 5 miles of jogging, and 2 miles of walking. This final slow gait allows the horse to "cool down" both mentally and physically. Strength and cardiovascular fitness will steadily increase. The horse should be able to jog 5 miles over flat ground with no noticeable signs of fatigue at the end of this phase. The horse is worked on alternate days with "off" days used for any remaining mental issues and for physical recovery. If the horse seems dull or listless during the scheduled work, two days "off" may be required between works. The goal is to avoid overtraining. We want the horse to gain fitness without acting worn out and "beat up". When the horse reaches that degree of fitness, it is ready to begin cantering or galloping.

Level 3

Week 9 Goal: Introduce Exercise at the Gallop, Jog Miles, and Work on Confidence

The horse has entered the final stage of establishing a foundation. The trainer will introduce galloping to the routine. Galloping will build strength but it will also develop the cardiovascular system in a way that jogging cannot do. This level of exercise will elevate the horse's heart rate and increase his demand for oxygen. Galloping will at first consist of a series of short intervals that will be gradually lengthened over time. After a warm up period of walking, ideally including some hill work, the horse is asked to jog for approximately one mile. Then, the pace is moved up to a slow canter for 1/8 of a mile. At that point, the horse is allowed to settle back into a jog – a "down-transition". This process is repeated four times to give a total work of a 5-mile jog interspersed with five, 1/8-mile gallops. The total length of the work will then be 5 and 5/8 miles. The horse is allowed to walk 1-2 miles to cool down mentally and physically. We are training the nervous system and making the horse comfortable and confident covering ground at the gallop during this time. By repeating the task multiple times i.e. asking the horse to travel at the gallop, the transition to this gait will not produce mental stress or anxiety. Again, the work is performed on an alternate day basis. It is important to work on confidence on the off day. When a horse encounters stimuli or obstacles at a faster pace, the likelihood of its spooking or bolting is greatly increased. It is important at this stage of conditioning for the horse to experience as many different training facilities as is logistically feasible. This will make unfamiliar surroundings less stressful as time passes.

Weeks 10-12 Goal: Increase Length of Gallop Intervals and Work on Confidence

The distance of the gallop interval is increased by 1/8 of a mile each week and the length of the jog is decreased by 1/8 mile until the horse is alternating a 1/2-mile jog with a 1/2-mile gallop therefore completing a total of 5 miles. Warm up and cool down are similar to week nine. If the horse has successfully completed this 12-week strategy, this work should not produce any noticeable signs of fatigue. The pulse of the horse should return to 60 beats/min or less within 15 minutes after completion of the work.

Summary: This 12-week strategy is designed to serve as a guide (see Figure 1). It will allow a trainer to formulate a conditioning strategy to fit a particular horse in a given facility. No conditioning program is appropriate for every horse. In fact, the above strategy will probably have to be modified somewhat for each individual animal. Completion of this strategy will provide a foundation for a horse that will allow it to be conditioned for the discipline in which it will compete. The horse will also be adequately desensitized to external stimuli so that additional stress will not stop or slow progress.

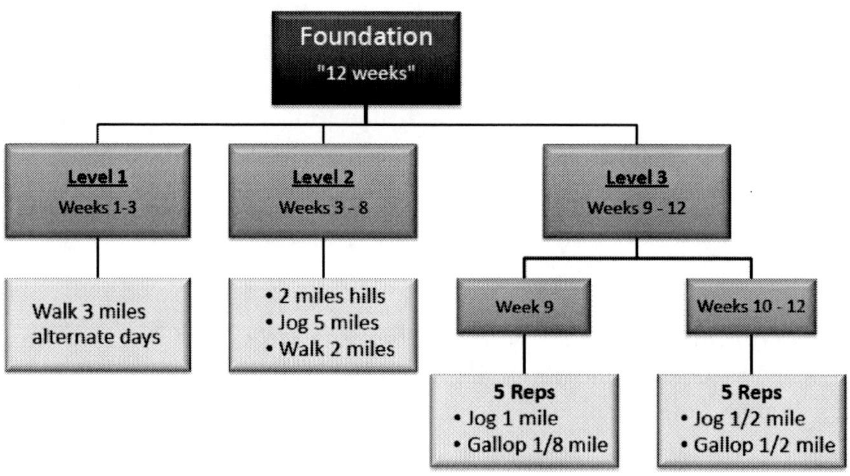

Figure 1.

STRATEGY FOR CONDITIONING TO BEGIN COMPETITION

Once a foundation has been firmly established, a strategy can be designed for a specific discipline. Due to the vast spectrum of equine disciplines and the variation in individual ability, it is difficult to prescribe generic conditioning strategies that will be universally applicable. It is at this stage that the advanced forms of conditioning are initiated. These include strength, speed, stamina, and plyometrics. Each of these is described in detail in this chapter. In all forms of advanced conditioning, the 10% rule should be employed. In its simplest form, this rule states that no more than a 10% alteration is allowed in the frequency (repetitions), intensity (amount of resistance of each repetition), or time (rest between sets of exertion) between conditioning days.

Strategy for Reconditioning to Return to Competition after an Injury

There are important considerations in designing a conditioning strategy that will enable a horse to re-enter competition after an injury has been rehabilitated. After a horse has gone through a conditioning program and competed in a given discipline, many of the steps in the basic conditioning strategy are no longer necessary. With these individuals, many of the mental issues present in the novice horse are not as evident. These issues can never be ignored but they do not require the same amount of time devoted to a novice horse. The primary goal now is to design a strategy that will allow re-entry into competition without re-injury. As with human athletic endeavors, all equine disciplines have their unique requirements for conditioning. Some place a heavy emphasis on speed while others are dependent on stamina, and still others require power. After a horse has recovered from an injury and has successfully regained a fitness level consistent with level three of the basic conditioning strategy, specific forms of conditioning can be utilized to enable reentry into competition. The forms of specialized conditioning described in this chapter must be carefully organized around not only the discipline but also the individual horse. The 10% rule applies here as it did for horses entering competition for the first time.

Advanced Conditioning: Strength, Speed, Endurance, and Plyometrics (see Figure 10).

Strength

This is an aspect of physical conditioning that has been emphasized in human athletics since the beginning of time. In the past few decades, strength has become recognized as a key factor in preventing injury in all forms of athletic endeavor. Some athletic endeavors, both human and equine, depend more on strength than others do. Strength is key to long-term participation in any athletic event however. Put in the simplest terms, a strong athlete is a durable athlete. In order to develop strength-building strategies for horses, we will examine some of the most recent theories and practices utilized in human athletics.

The extraordinary performances seen in sports today are a function of genetic inheritance, fine-tuned skills, and physical conditioning. In order to excel, the athlete must bring to his or her sport an entire strategy. The strategy is enhanced through physical conditioning and by an established fitness base. Thus, the basis for performance in elite competition is not a single factor, but rather a combination of many factors coming together to peak on a specific date.

Developing a sports-fitness/strength base is important for both the performance and the health of the athlete. A comprehensive program, which addresses every aspect of the athlete's physical and mental state, is critical to success. The development of a strength base at the beginning of an athlete's training cycle will help with many aspects of his/her development. The base will lead to greater performance gains and quicker return to competition should injury occur. One of the most common training concepts, which lends to this type of success is called "linear periodization". Linear periodization, in simple terms, is a training cycle that provides a highly organized strategy to bring the athlete to optimal performance levels at the right time. As an athlete moves through the training cycle, a base is established by starting with higher volume (number of repetitions) and lower intensity (e. g., amount of weight lifted). The volume will be reduced and the intensity will be elevated as the training cycle progresses allowing for more intense training to be initiated. Periodization is typically used in resistance training programs but any conditioning program can and should be periodized to provide necessary variation in exercise stimulus and recovery periods.

The concept of linear periodization can and should definitely be applied to strength training in horses. Strategies based on the periodization concept are much less prone to result in injury to a rehabilitating horse. Therefore, it is imperative that periodization be incorporated into controlled exercises protocols. From a practical standpoint, it is somewhat harder to perform resistance training exercise for horses than for humans. Horses cannot "lift weights" in the traditional sense. This does not mean that resistance training cannot be performed and appropriate training strategies devised. The three strength training modalities that can be utilized are hill repeats, steps, and sand.

Hills

Controlled exercise performed on inclines is an excellent way to increase strength, "hill work" is safe and effective when a periodization strategy is used (Figure 2 & 3). Research has shown that exercise performed on an incline produces more quadriceps shortening than when performed on a flat surface. This form of muscle isolation is necessary to achieve maximal gains in strength of particular muscle groups. The advantageous aspect of hill work is that it can be carefully controlled in terms of incline, speed, number of repetitions, and distance. As strength increases, all of these factors can be increased in a periodized manner i.e. fewer repetitions of longer, steeper hills at a faster pace with less rest in between hills.

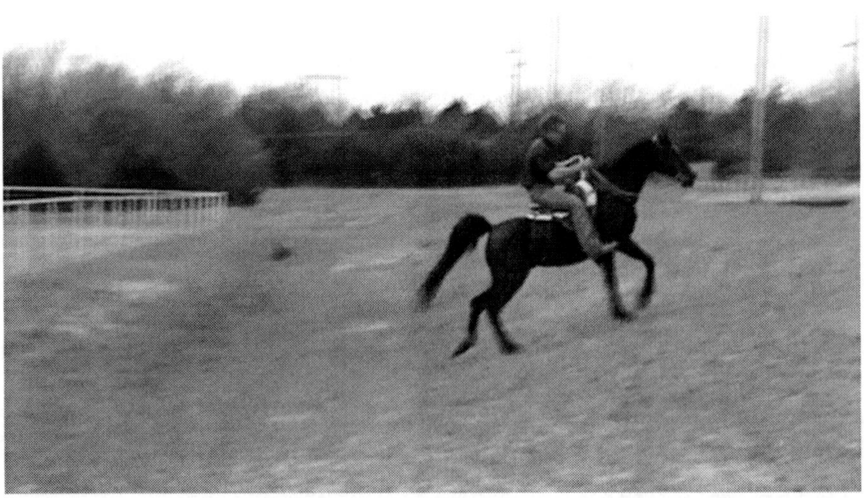

Figure 2.

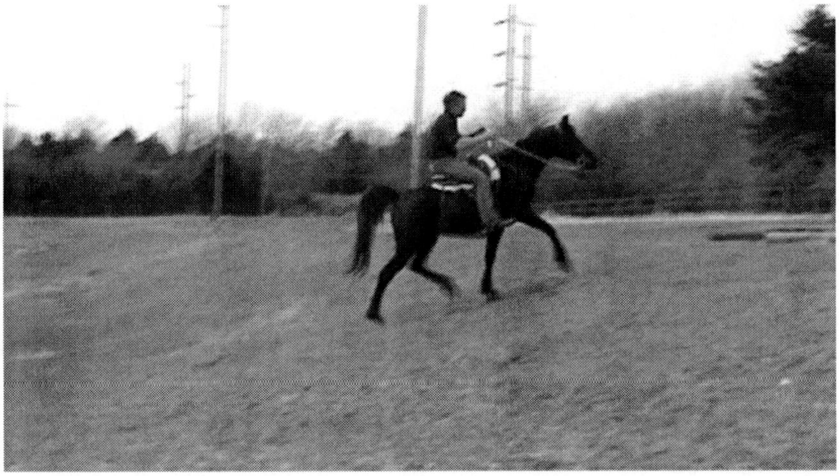

Figure 3.

Steps

Step work is a more advanced form of resistance training than hill work. The primary difference between working on steps versus working on a hill is that steps do not allow for shortening of the stride as fatigue increases (Figure 4, 5, 6, 7, 8, & 9). The stride length must stay the same or the individual will stumble and fall. In order to maintain speed, the muscles must work harder because the stride cannot be shortened. This is a more difficult form of resistance training than are hills. This form of controlled exercise is actually more easily periodized than hill work because it is easier to count repetitions. In this case, step work can begin at a very slow pace and a low number of repetitions. The speed (pace) and number of repetitions are increased only to a point at which the level of fatigue is relatively constant. In other words, it will take more and more repetitions to produce the same level of fatigue that was present on initial training sessions. This methodology will increase strength while minimizing the risk of injury. NOTE: If for logistical reasons steps are unobtainable, cavalettis can be substituted for steps.

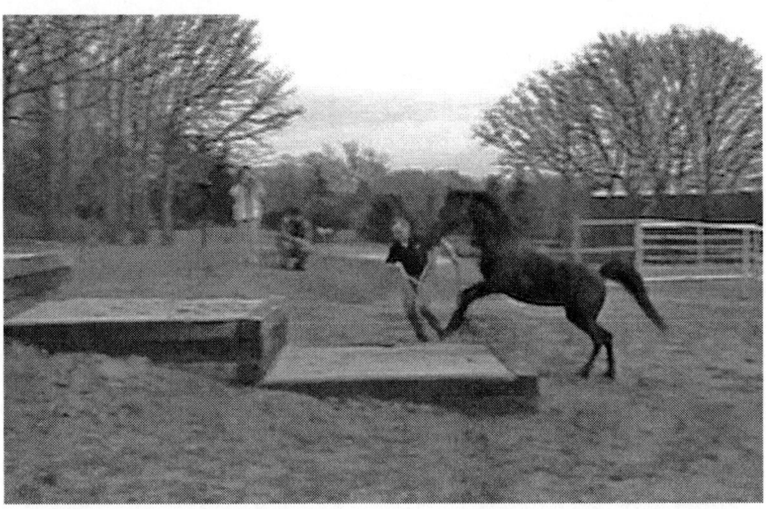

Figure 4.

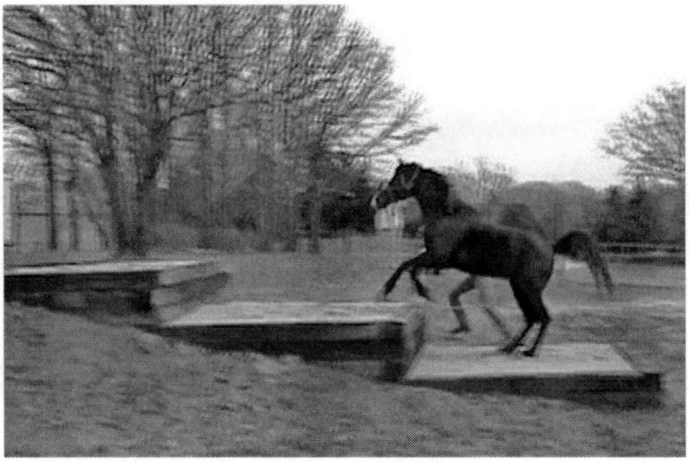

Figure 5.

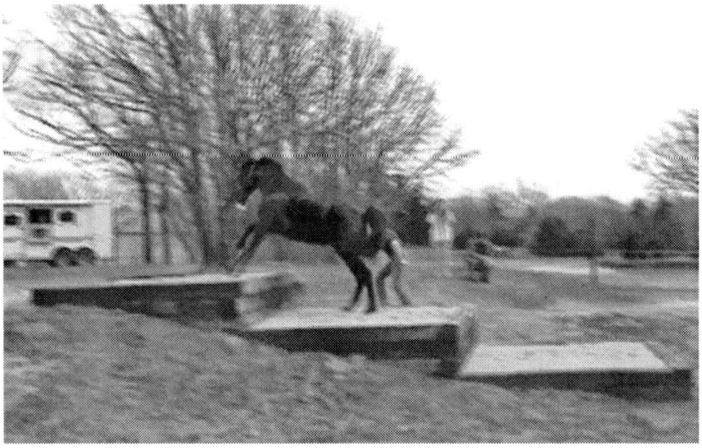

Figure 6.

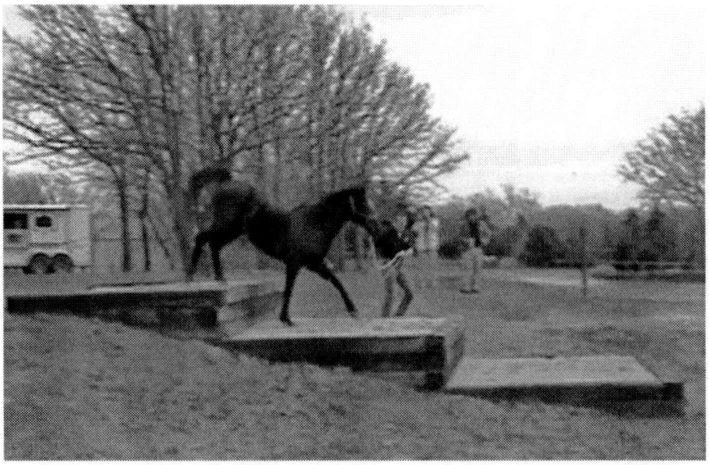

Figure 7.

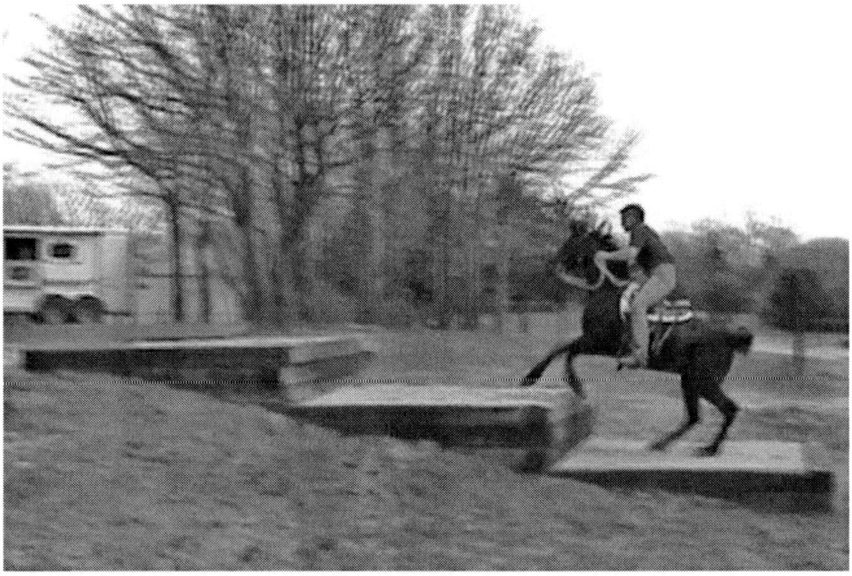

Figure 8.

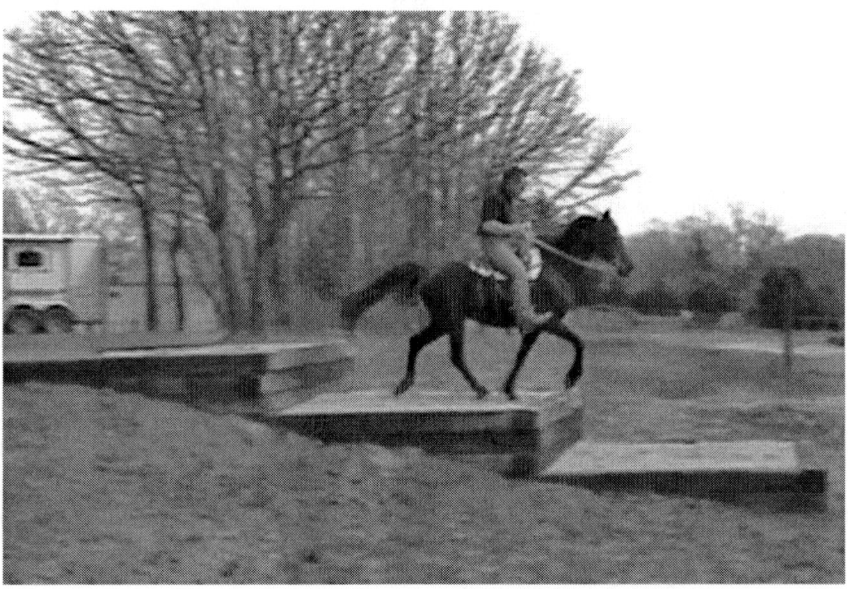

Figure 9.

Sand

Controlled exercise performed in sand represents a form of resistance training that is safe and can be easily periodized. Ridden exercise performed in sand increases the exertion level at all gaits and is therefore a way to increase muscular effort without increasing speed. It should be noted by those who train regularly in sand, what a difference a small variation in depth can make in the amount of effort required of the horse. The exertion can be increased by increasing the depth of sand, speed of gait, and distance at various gaits. As strength (fitness) increases, speed can be increased without increasing exertion or risk of injury.

Speed

Speed is a component of almost all forms of equine athletic endeavor. Many athletic events are won or lost by seconds or fractions of seconds. In horses, as in humans, speed is determined largely by genetics and muscle physiology. Although some improvement can be achieved it cannot be improved upon to the extent that strength and stamina can. What conditioning can achieve is to train an athlete to perform at his/her maximum speed without becoming injured. The majority of all injuries in both equine and human athletics are in some way related to speed. We must therefore condition horses and humans to perform at speed to allow musculoskeletal and nervous system adaptations to occur. Human athletes undergo extensive speed training that involves performing various drills as rapidly as possible. We know that to increase speed there are two components that must be addressed: One is the athlete's stride length (the distance between strides), the other being the stride frequency (the time interval between strides). When working on stride length, it is first necessary to increase flexibility of the musculature. Power applied at the point of contact with the ground is later developed by strength training and plyometrics. The stride frequency is addressed by enhancing the ability of the central nervous system to get the muscle to fire and a faster than normal rate. This can be achieved by over-speed training, e.g.downhill running, and towing.

Speed can be further specialized into four components: start speed, acceleration, maximum speed, and deceleration. Different athletic events require different combinations of these components. Each of these must be considered or emphasized depending on an athlete's specific requirements for a given competitive event.

In order to return a horse to competition, speed must be introduced into the rehabilitation strategy gradually. Logically, it should follow controlled strength training to minimize the risk of re-injury. Speed should be introduced in the form of sub-maximal increments to allow motor coordination to adapt (i.e., the athlete must relearn to functioning at speed). Speed work should not produce excessive fatigue. Rather, it should be introduced in such a way that exertion does not exceed the fitness level of an individual athlete. Also it should not exceed the ability of the body to recover effectively from each speed or high intensity training session. There are no set numbers that can be applied to the various equine disciplines. In Thoroughbred racing, tolerance of speed is usually introduced in 1/8 mile increments striving to perform each unit in approximately 12 seconds. Increments are gradually increased with a set goal of 5/8 mile in 60 seconds. The other equine disciplines are not as well standardized and there are no set measures of maximal speed. However, unlike thoroughbred racing, most other equine disciplines do not require the horse to perform at maximal speed.

Stamina

Stamina as it applies to athletics is the ability to delay the onset of fatigue. A tired athlete is not only less likely to win but he/she is much more prone to injury. As muscles of the appendicular skeleton fatigue the diarthrodial joints are more likely to become hyperextended. This condition contributes to a large proportion of articular and periarticular injuries. The axial musculature can also fatigue leading to increased strain of the ligamentous components of the sacro-iliac joint with subsequent sprain and luxation, and possible injury to neural elements. Furthermore, a tired athlete has decreased ability to perform learned motor skills and is more likely to make a misstep over uneven terrain or to negotiate a jump or other obstacle poorly. Simply put – appropriate conditioning will delay the onset of "rubber-leggedness" that greatly increases the likelihood of injury.

In humans, extensive strategies have been developed over the past 50 years to augment stamina. In the past, athletes have often simply "played themselves into shape". Only recently, has the concept of year-round training following a periodization strategy been embraced. Gradually, athletes and coaches have begun to attribute the success of certain individuals and teams to their intense physical conditioning off the field. It is now generally accepted that such conditioning provides that much-needed "edge" in competition.

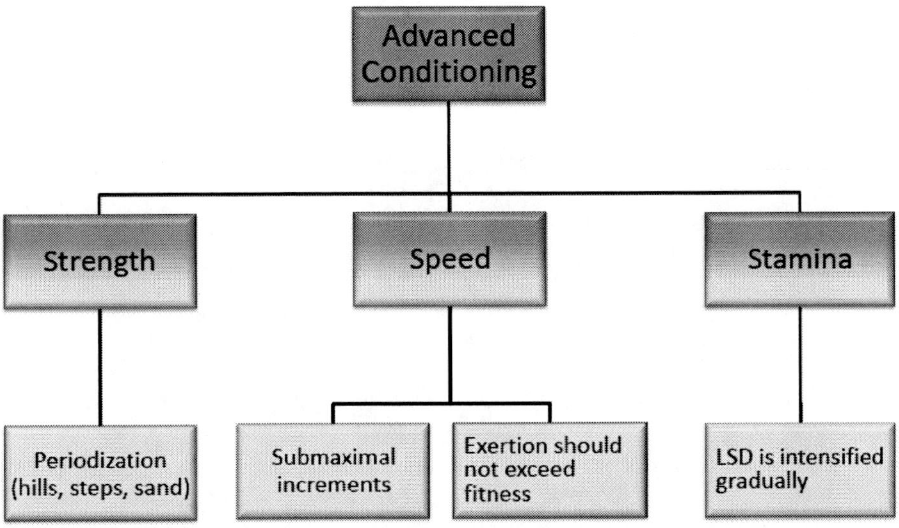

Figure 10.

Equine sports disciplines require stamina in varying degrees. Stamina cannot be acquired rapidly. It is the most time consuming aspect of physical conditioning. The greater the level of stamina required, the longer it takes to acquire. The basis for the development of stamina is long, slow distance work similar to that described in the foundation portion of this chapter. That foundation "layer" is taken to a higher level, and distance is added to the training strategy in gradual increments. When a horse can cover a given distance easily, speed is also increased gradually. Distance and speed are increased alternately. The horse is never asked to exceed a given distance at a comfortable (non-fatiguing) speed. As fitness increases, both distance and speed will increase, i.e., a given horse will be able to travel farther and faster without fatigue. Unlike strength and speed that can be acquired in a period of several months, a high level of stamina can take 2-3 years to develop. Although ultimate stamina is strongly influenced by body type and breed (genetics), any sound horse can develop a high level of stamina with an appropriate conditioning strategy. This is one area where periodization takes on a more gradual and continuous application, i.e., the athlete is subjected to increasingly more demanding exercise without a sudden transition between levels of speed and distance.

Plyometrics

Plyometrics is a form of exercise designed to enable a muscle to reach maximal strength as rapidly as possible. In the simplest of terms it is the combination of strength and speed that is referred to as power. This form of athletic capability is part of all equine disciplines in varying degrees. It is essential that any advanced equine conditioning program include some form of plyometrics. There are two important aspects of equine plyometric conditioning that must be considered. First, it is a very advanced form of controlled exercise because it combines speed and strength. As such it carries a high risk of causing re-injury and must be advanced cautiously Second, plyometrics are technically more difficult to perform than the other forms of specialized conditioning because it involves a forceful and precise motor act performed repeatedly as rapidly as possible (Figure 11, 12, & 13).

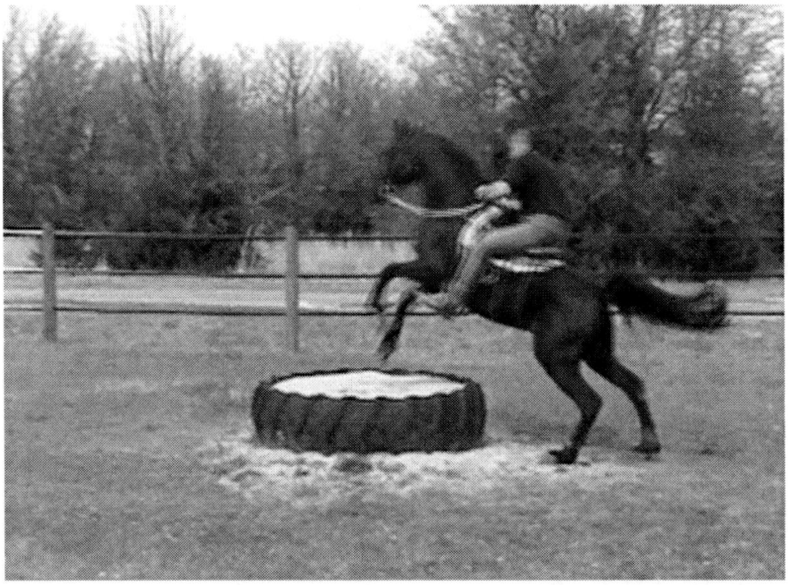

Figure 11.

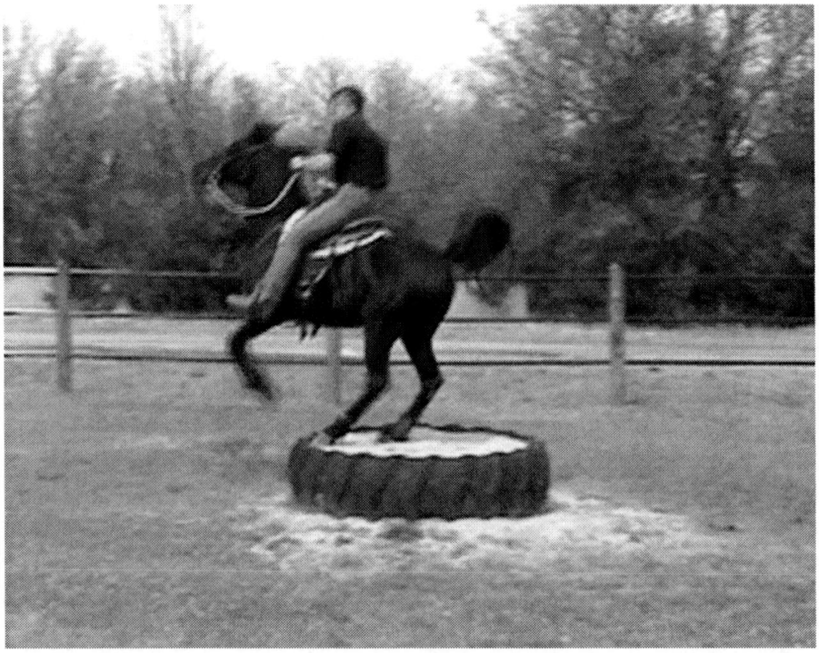

Figure 12.

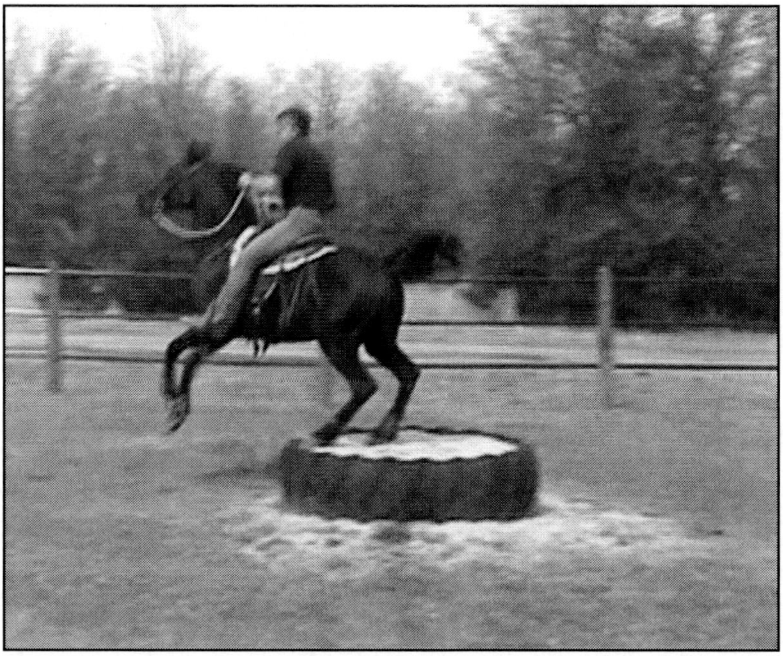

Figure 13.

The skill of the exercise rider and the motor skill (training) of the horse are therefore essential components of any form of plyometric conditioning program (Figures 14, 15, 16, & 17).

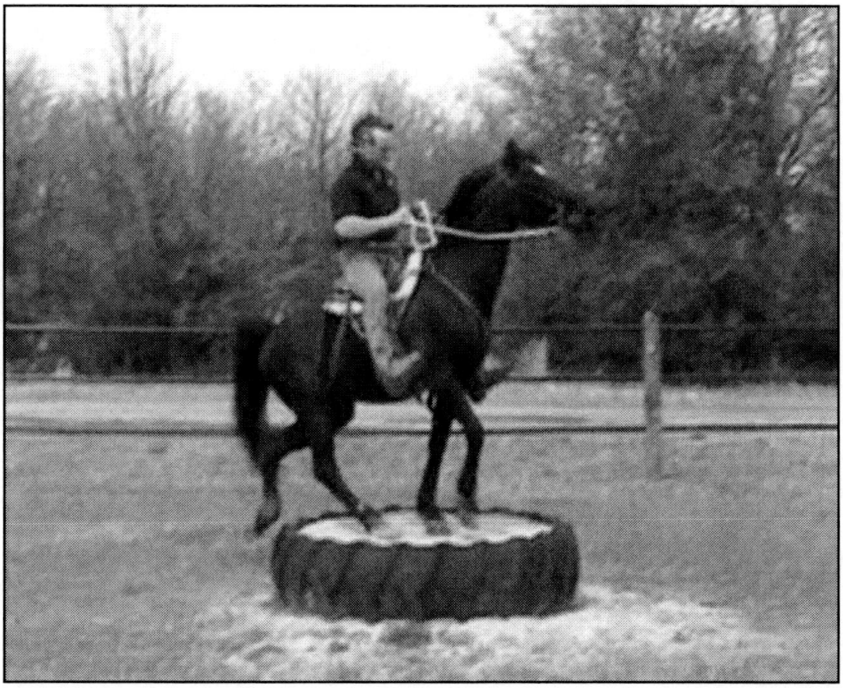

Figure 14.

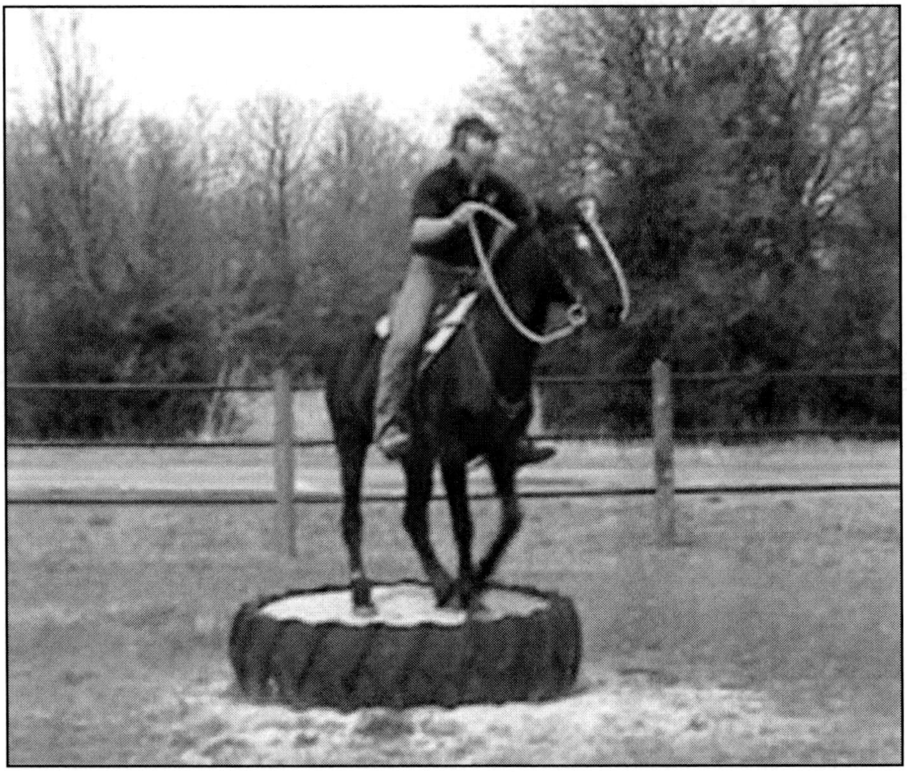

Figure 15.

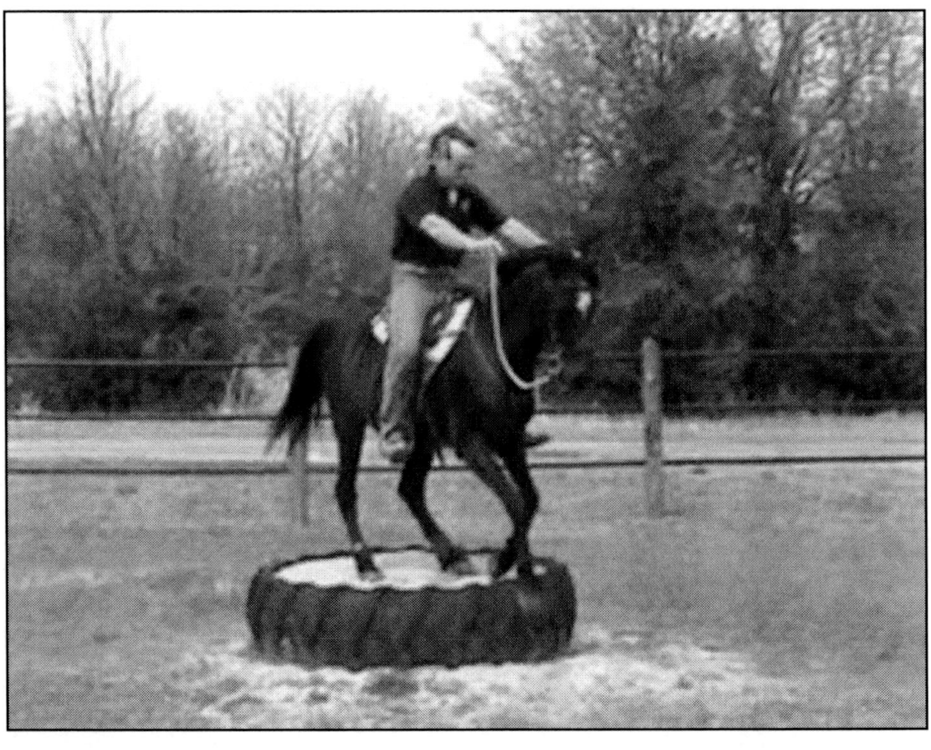

Figure 16.

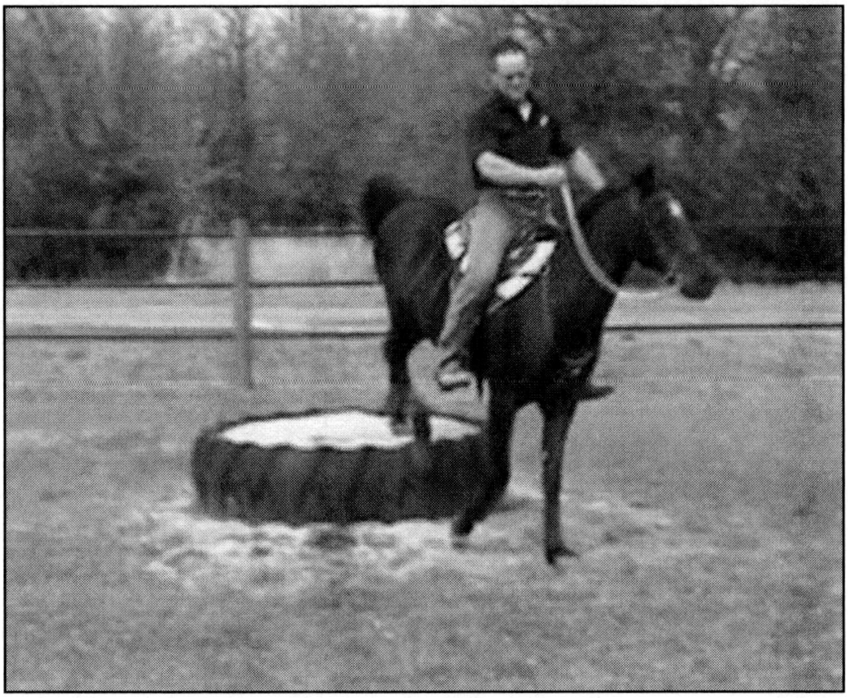

Figure 17.

It is important that neither one of these components is exceeded because this will likely result in re-injury or even in the creation of a new one. Examples of equine plyometric training strategies include all the components of the strength conditioning program, e. g., hills, steps, and sand. These components are utilized in a manner that involves rapid repetition. As the conditioning strategy progresses the number of repetitions increases for a given time allotment – simply put: the horse performs more repetitions in less time. This training result is a function of less time required to perform each repetition and less time between repetitions.

MAINTENANCE OF PHYSICAL CONDITION

Once a horse has been rehabilitated to the point of returning to competition, trainers should not discard the overall conditioning schedule that was utilized in the process. In fact, overall fitness level must be maintained to prevent recurrence of the original injury or the development of another one if the horse is to remain in competition. It is a common misconception that the mere act of competing in a given discipline will keep a horse fit enough to prevent overexertion and subsequent injury. In most equine disciplines, the actual act of competing is not enough of a physiologic challenge to result in a high level of fitness. Repeated competitive events increase the probability of injury to musculoskeletal structures due to loads and strain rates that may exceed physiologic limits. Therefore, a maintenance fitness regime is indicated for any horse that competes. The question becomes: How much is enough, and how much is too much? Due to the wide variety of equine disciplines these questions are not easily answered. There are, however, some general considerations that are valid regardless of discipline:

1) A reasonable level of cardiovascular fitness must be maintained. Obviously, the more physically demanding the discipline, the more important this becomes. Between competitions, the horse must be asked to exert itself in a way that will prevent loss of cardiovascular fitness.
2) Strength training will reduce the risk of injury, regardless of discipline. This is based on the premise expressed earlier in this chapter that a strong athlete is a durable one. Strength training can be incorporated into a routine weekly strategy.
3) Speed work is an essential part of a fitness program. If the horse is not asked to perform at speed *between* competitions it will lack the confidence and the motor skill to perform at speed *during* competition. Speed is not only dangerous but it is also useless without control. An animal that works at speed only during competition is more prone to injury from uncontrolled movements, the consequences of which are exaggerated by fatigue.
4) The mental and emotional aspects of training a horse must never be overlooked. Incessant repetition of the same task produces a horse with a robot-like personality, often associated with resentment and dysfunctional behavior patterns. Variation in training strategies will help keep the horse alert, enthusiastic, and interested in its work.

Conclusion

Controlled exercise is the basis for preparation for competition. It is also a fundamental component of rehabilitation. Controlled exercise strategies are initiated by establishing a foundation of both cardiovascular and musculoskeletal fitness. This foundation is then refined to include varying degrees of strength, speed, stamina, and plyometrics. The actual requirement of each of these components is dependent upon the individual and the discipline of the individual. Throughout this chapter, the mental and emotional aspects of controlled exercise strategies were emphasized because it is often these aspects that represent the limiting factors in an individual's rate of advancement.

References

[1] Burch PM, Bower A. *Training thoroughbred horses*. Menasha, WI: R. Meerdink Co.; 1992.

[2] Baechle TR, Earle RW. *Essentials of strength training and conditioning*. 3rd ed. Champaign, IL: Human Kinetics; 2008.

[3] Bompa TO, Bompa TO. *Periodization: Theory and methodology of training*. 4th ed. Champaign, IL: Human Kinetics; 1999.

[4] Clayton HM. *Conditioning sport horses*. Saskatoon: Sport Horse Publications; 1991.

[5] Clayton HM. *The dynamic horse : a biomechanical guide to equine movement and performance*. Mason, MI: Sport Horse Publications; 2004.

[6] Garrard K, Nolan LE. *Nolans system for training cavalry horses*. New York: D. Van Nostrand; 1862.

[7] Kraemer WJ, Fleck SJ. *Optimizing strength training: Designing nonlinear periodization workouts*. Champaign, IL: Human Kinetics; 2007.

[8] Marlin D, Nankervis KJ. *Equine exercise physiology*. Malden, MA: Blackwell Science; 2002.

[9] *Military-Info. Cavalry (Horse Mounted).* 2009 July 1. Available from: http://www.military-info.com/mphoto/p011.htm.

In: Rehabilitating the Athletic Horse
Editors: H. W. Jann et al., pp. 179-201
ISBN: 978-1-678-1-60876-672-7

Chapter 9

PSYCHOLOGICAL ASPECTS OF REHABILITATION

Cassie Smith[1], Robert M. Miller[2] and Pat Parelli[3]
[1]http://home.earthlink.net/~outdoorlady/, Oklahoma City, Oklahoma, USA
[2]DVM, Robert M Miller Communications, Truckee, California, USA
[3]Parelli Natural Horsemanship, Inc., Pagosa Springs, Colorado, USA

ABSTRACT

The goal of this chapter is to increase awareness of the need for changes in how we view the success or failure of rehabilitation. By considering the psychological aspects of rehabilitation as well as surgery, wound treatment, and physical rehabilitation we begin treating each patient more thoroughly. We will increase safety for horses and humans, reduce possible litigation for injuries occurring during rehabilitation, improve relations with clients and create confidence and assurance that we are treating someone's prized possession with the dignity, respect and care they deserve.

The mental and emotional aspects of rehabilitation are too often underemphasized or completely neglected. Horses in long term confinement situations often develop dysfunctional behavior patterns that can be difficult if not impossible to correct. This chapter is divided into four segments: 1) a typical case history 2) an explanation of why the mental and emotional aspects of equine veterinary care and rehabilitation can be problematic 3) specific mental and emotional aspects that must be considered during rehabilitation 4) and recommendations for improved care and increased success before, during and after the rehabilitation process occurs.

INTRODUCTION

CASE HISTORY ZIP: CASSIE SMITH

A 6 month old Quarter Horse filly sustained a 23 inch long laceration in the left axillary region that resulted from straddling a barbed wire fence. The laceration was 18 inches deep but did not disrupt the major neurovascular components of the axillary region. This wound required 9 months to heal during which time there was continuous veterinary care and the filly was confined to stall for 3½ months. Following the time required for the wound to heal a progressive personality change developed. The filly became very fearful and distrusting of humans and unfamiliar situations. Over the next three years of life these personality problems regressed to the point that the filly was dangerous to interact with. In fact, she would strike, kick, and bite any stranger or veterinarian that approached her. This behavior was not manifested with the owner.

A slow and progressive desensitization and confidence building process was initiated that allowed this mare to successfully regain trust in strangers and veterinarians. She regained her naturally trusting personality and was no longer a threat to humans. Without this careful reprogramming process this mare would probably never have been resocialized and have a normal life. The lesson learned from this case is that this dysfunctional behavior could have been avoided if she would have been exposed to people and situations during rehabilitation that were positive and confidence building. Instead, during her entire rehabilitation period in the very early months and years of her life, all strangers represented an ongoing predatorial threat. She had never known a stranger that did not hurt her in some way. It should be noted that during the procedures the filly remained calm and cooperative without extreme restraint. Her natural trusting personality and willingness to cooperate lulled the caregivers into ignoring the filly's pain and stress levels. This ***lack of observation*** led to behavior that would not have been as pronounced or extreme had routine procedures and daily interaction been handled in a different manner.

There are many horses that develop behavioral problems from prolonged confinement and continual unpleasant interaction with humans. Zip was fortunate because her behavioral issues were recognized as learned responses and attitudes resulting from a very abnormal and totally stressful environment. She was slowly and skillfully allowed to work through them until they had become totally resolved. Many horses are not that fortunate and these kinds of behavioral problems eventually become worse until the horse never becomes a useful animal or even worse is destroyed.

WHY DO HORSES MAKE SUCH DIFFICULT PATIENTS? ROBERT M. MILLER DVM

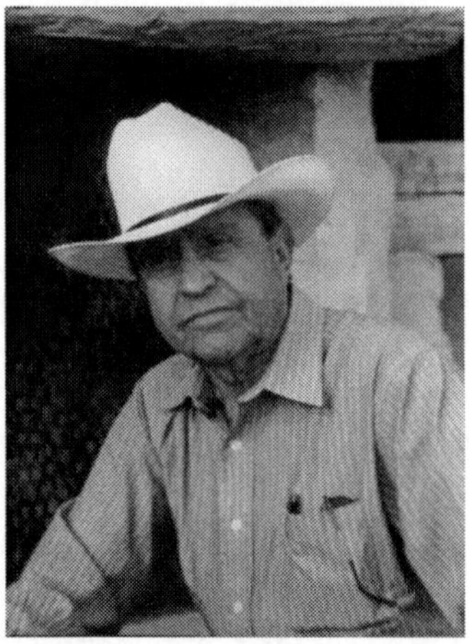

Not all horses are difficult patients. Some are remarkably cooperative, but they are exceptional. We are all too familiar with successful equine athletes that suffered a serious injury which with state of the art medical technology, could have survived and had a wonderful life, but because they were refractory and uncooperative, they ended up with euthanasia.

In order to understand why most horses are intolerant of confinement, isolation and the boredom of post-traumatic or post-surgical rehabilitation, we must understand the basic genetically predetermined behavior of the species.

The horse is a prey species. In the wild state it is hunted by voracious predatory species. Inhabitants of the grasslands, and not possessing the lethal weaponry of other herbivorous prey species such as the horns of a rhinoceros or buffalo, or the tusks of a hippopotamus or elephant, the horse is dependent upon flight to survive. The efficacy of this speaks for itself. Horses have been around for more than fifty million years.

It should be understood that horses are not innately afraid of predators. They fear predatory behavior. Thus the stalk and the charge precipitate flight in the horse. That's why stationary unfamiliar objects or a stalking posture frighten the horse. It is also why any unfamiliar movement towards the horse is interpreted as intimidation, and stimulates the flight response. Conversely, predators do not retreat, so movement of a novel stimulus away from a horse is reassuring.

We have all seen, on television, scenes of zebra, for example, peacefully grazing within sight of lions in repose. But, let the cats begin their stalk, and flight is precipitated.

The horse is also a group species living in bands of varying size. In nature, the horse is never alone.

Because the horse has depended on flight as its primary survival behavior for so many millions of years, it has evolved certain qualities which enhance the flight response:

1) It is an extremely perceptive species. It's senses quickly detect stimuli to which we humans may be oblivious.
2) It has remarkably fast reaction time, a necessity in an animal which must sprint away from danger. This reaction time is an asset to humans, who have domesticated the horse and directed its flight response down the racetrack, into the harness collar, over fences, after cattle, around barrels and into a cavalry charge. This very fast reaction time also accounts for the frequency with which horses injure humans or themselves.
3) It is an extremely fast learner. The slow learners did not survive to reproduce. Moreover, horses remember what they have learned. The horse is the fastest learner and has the best memory of any domesticated animal.

All of the above serve to make the horse a poor patient, but there is hope. Horses can be de-sensitized (Figure 2) to frightening stimuli, no matter how severe, with remarkable speed, if we know how to do it, and so long as these frightening stimuli are not painful. How this will be accomplished will be discussed later by my co-authors.

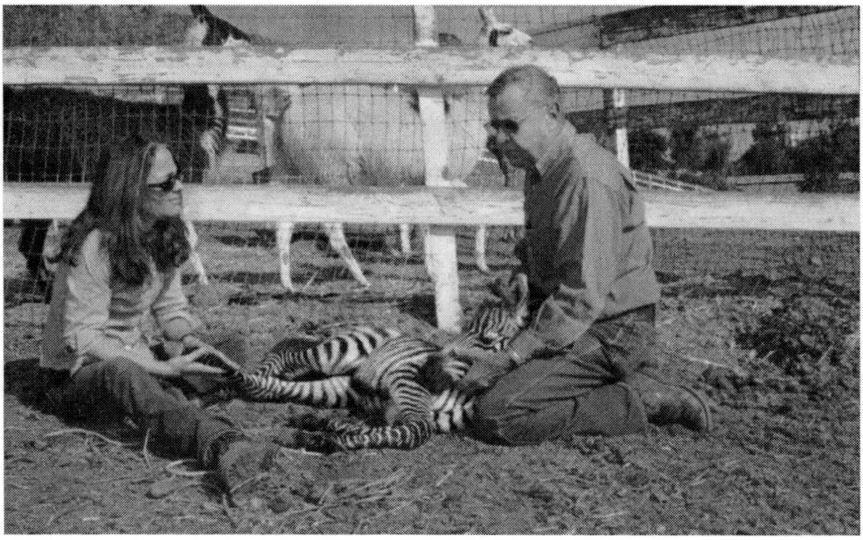

Figure 2.

Moreover, the horse being a group species seeks leadership. Even an alpha – a naturally dominant leader – can be led, and in horses the dominance hierarchy is principally established by the leader controlling the movement of its peers.

If we compare a horse, as a patient, to a dog or cat, it is easy to understand the difficulties involved in the equine rehabilitation. Dogs and cats are carnivores. In nature they hunt, gorge, and then lie around until hunger prompts them to hunt again. They are comfortable in dens, or confined spaces.

Horses in the wild graze for ten to as much as eighteen hours a day. Their stomachs are never full and are never empty. They relish open space where they can see their mates, or an approaching enemy. Horse can sleep standing up, and with their eyes open. Confined spaces are threatening to horses. They are naturally claustrophobic. Considering all of the above, it is easy to understand why horses, especially of athletic bloodlines are intolerant of confining box stalls, are disturbed when isolated from other individuals, are extremely uncomfortable with anything that limits their mobility such as casts, neck cradles, body slings, etc.

Moreover, people constantly coming around with things that the horse is unfamiliar with, that smell strange, look strange, make strange sounds, and feel strange and are often painful, create a powerful desire to be somewhere else.

If we humans are uncomfortable when we are hospitalized, if dogs or cats are unhappy, how much worse must it be for a horse?

Thus several factors which are typical during rehabilitation contribute to the horse so frequently being an unhappy and uncooperative patient. Again, these are: isolation, boredom, confinement, immobility, and pain.

However, one other factor even more than those listed above, is a major cause of difficulty, and that is past experience. Keeping in mind how perceptive horses are, their keen senses, and how persistent their memory, every significant memory determines how a horse will react to a new environment and unfamiliar stimuli. Moreover, horses categorize memorized experiences into A- things to run away from OR B – Things to accept.

Depending upon how various experiences in life have been presented, horses can decide that such innocuous things such as electric clippers, plastic, horse trailers, veterinarians, and wet spots on the ground are things to run away from.

Conversely, using appropriate techniques, horses can be taught to peacefully tolerate, cannon fire, llamas, marching bands, flags and fire engines.

It is also significant that this learning begins at birth. Horses are a precocial species, like so many other prey animals, able to follow their dam or the herd soon after birth.

Unlike altricial species, such as dogs, cats, bears, or humans, foals are neurologically mature at birth. All of their senses are fully functional. Most important, their imprinting period is immediately post partum, and their critical learning times are all crowded into the first days of life.

Therefore, how newborn foals are handled and what they experience is a major factor in determining their behavior later in life. This is true of all species, but in the case of altricial species, these critical learning periods are delayed. (Approx. one to four months of age in the dog and much later and much longer in humans.)

Proper handling of newborn foals, a technique I discovered in 1959, can prepare foals for all sorts of experiences, including veterinary procedures, farriery, and hospitalization techniques, after maturity. Conversely, traumatic handling and events will never be forgotten.

Because new born foals learn so fast and so lastingly, it is essential that any learning presented at this age be skillfully and correctly done.

Obviously, the armamentarium of behavior modifying drugs at our disposal today, are extremely useful in minimizing problems during rehabilitation. None of these drugs were available when I began practice in 1956. However, it is a mistake to believe that these drugs lessen the importance of handling horses correctly. The first experience, of any kind, at any age will be remembered by the horse and will determine future response to the same stimulus. Yes, undesirable behavior can be mitigated. Fearful responses can be placated. Fight or flight responses can be subdued. But it's much better, much safer, and takes less time to teach young horses not to be fearful and to be respectful and cooperative.

My Thoughts on Postsurgical Rehab
Robert M. Miller, DVM

In recent times the popular press has exploited two cases of racetrack trauma to exceptional Thoroughbred racehorses. The first of these was "Ruffian". After being skillfully operated, her agitation post surgically led to her demise.

The second case that brought worldwide attention was "Barbaro". Although complications eventually led to his euthanasia, Barbaro was widely acclaimed as a model patient, remarkably gentle and accepting of the myriad daily procedures entailed in his post surgical recovery.

A clue to "Barbaro's" cooperative patient status is revealed in the book Barbaro, the horse's biography. In the opening chapter it is revealed that his birth involved a complex dystocia, caused by a difficult malpositioning during parturition. This necessitated extensive manipulation and post delivery handling.

It was a series of three such dystocias in May of 1959 that led me to develop my foal imprinting regimen. Although I had always been warned to minimize handling of the newborn foal because it would contribute to the foal growing up into a spoiled and disrespectful horse, that it would encourage the mare to reject the foal, and that it would cause the mare to be aggressive towards her postpartum human handlers, none of these things happened. What did happen was that these foals were exceptionally gentle, obviously remembered me when I saw them again many weeks later, accepted me willingly, and tolerated all sorts of handling.

I was familiar with the studies Konrad Lorenz had done in Europe with newly hatched goslings, which led him to the concept of "imprinting." I concluded that extensive immediate postpartum handling of foals would result in them being "imprinted" by their handlers. After experimenting with my own foals and developing a ritualized training regimen I became an advocate for "imprint training" of foals (Figure 3). Eventually books and videos on the method popularized the method which is now in use all over the world.

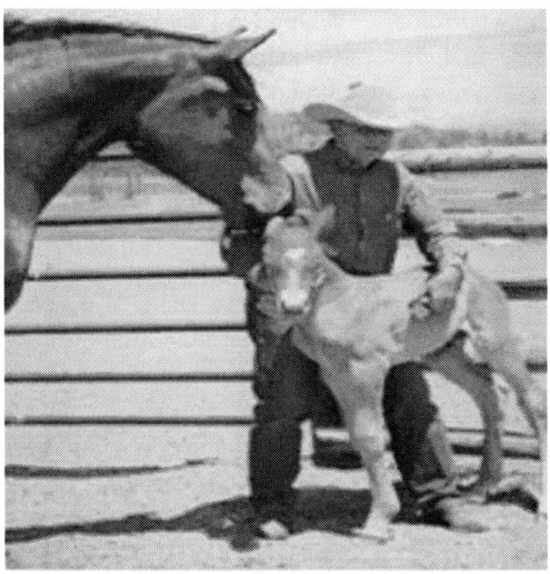

Figure 3.

Because I was a practicing veterinarian my principal goal was to produce gentle and cooperative patients. Indeed this was remarkably successful. Those farms which imprint trained their foals as I advocated had horses which were a pleasure to treat.

I cite the experience because as I list the rehabilitation suggestions which I have been asked to, which will hopefully minimize some of the post surgical problems which are so common, the first and most important thing I recommend is imprint training.

In more recent decades I have learned that training newborn foals enhances future learning ability and future performance. However my original motivation was to create cooperative patients, and this was successful for three decades before I retired from practice. We had entire farms of cooperative and accepting equine patients.

With this in mind I will list the things I believe can be done to minimize rehab problems:

1) Imprint Train every foal, but do it exactly as I recommend. It must be done correctly to obtain the desired results.
2) Do not isolate the patient. In an adjacent stall, provide a round-the-clock companion. This can be another horse, a pony, a burro or miniature donkey, or a goat. It should be protected with a stall of its own, but the separation between it and the patient should permit full visual contact as well as olfactory contact and tactile contact (through bars or a grill). Ideally the patient and the companion, if possible, should be allowed to bond for a few days prior to surgery.
3) If the patient is agitated or emotionally upset post operatively, many sedatives, tranquilizers and behavior modifying drugs are available for chronic use, but I recommend they be used in minimal dosages. We do not want soporific effects, or to interfere with musculoskeletal coordination or balance. One thing that should be tried is the mood ameliorating pheromones that have become recently available. They seem to have a calming effect.However if the horse is content, then I would avoid using any behavior modifying chemicals.
4) If possible, the horse should be trained with Parelli's Natural Horsemanship ground school techniques. If this were done previously it will do much to smooth rehab. If not, and it is feasible, some of this may be able to be done post operatively.
5) Most important, the handlers of the patient – the technicians, grooms, and the veterinarians should be schooled in Parelli's Natural Horsemanship techniques. We are not discussing horsemanship under saddle. We mean horsemanship on the ground.

How a stall is entered by a veterinarian, tech, groom or caregiver, their demeanor, and their knowledge of the art and science of horsemanship is virtually important as to whether or not rehabilitation will be successful.

"Bedside manner" is as vital to recuperation as is surgical expertise. The horse that is happy in the rehab stall, is unafraid of the handlers and is fond of them is glad to see them because they know how to get along with horses, has a better chance of a successful recovery. This is true for not only psychological and physiological reasons, but also for more mundane and practical reasons. These include:

1) Minimizing trauma to the horse
2) Minimizing trauma to the handlers (vets, grooms, and technicians)
3) Minimizing litigation, malpractice allegations, damage to the property, damage to costly equipment used for diagnostic and therapeutic purposes.
4) Improving client/hospital relations. The client is going to be favorably impressed if the horse is gentle and cooperative and treatment is as non-coercive, considerable, and humane as possible.

I can think of no better teacher to educate the horse and the medical personnel who handle the horse than Pat Parelli. If every horse were ground schooled via his methods and every veterinarian, veterinary technician, and hospital groom were skilled in his methods, it would greatly enhance postoperative rehabilitation.

BICEPS Concept Developed by Dr. Hank Jann DVM
Cassie Smith

For convenience, the mental and emotional aspects of rehabilitation have been grouped into six categories: Boredom, Isolation, Confinement, Environment, Pain, and Staff. The mnemonic device BICEPS can be used to remember these six concepts. Each of these must be considered when providing the optimal rehabilitation situation.

Pat Parelli, the world renowned natural horseman graciously offered his thoughts on the BICEPS concept of rehabilitation (Figure 4). His perspective concurs with Dr. Robert M. Miller's thoughts on this subject. It is clear that prior and proper preparation is the key to helping ensure a more likely positive outcome after a catastrophic injury requiring long term rehabilitation has occurred. Recognizing that this idea helps both horse and human leads us to believe that more emphasis should be placed on education and training of equine caregivers in the area of horsemanship. Additionally, properly preparing horses for interaction with humans and routine medical procedures should be promoted by all individuals who are in a position of providing care of any kind to horses.

The goal of this chapter is to create a sense of urgency to recognize that learning to become better horsemen is critical to the improved care of horses. Years of previous training, ideology, and methodology have resulted in an attitude of, "that is how we have always done it". By recognizing and accepting the new revolution towards a more natural approach to interacting with horses we reap an abundance of rewards. Horses and humans can develop relationships that lead to safer and more productive outcomes. Those who choose a career in working with horses are in a unique position to educate and/or make recommendations that will assist caregivers in treating and caring for the entire patient rather than just the injury.

Mental and Emotional Aspects of Rehabilitation
Pat Parelli

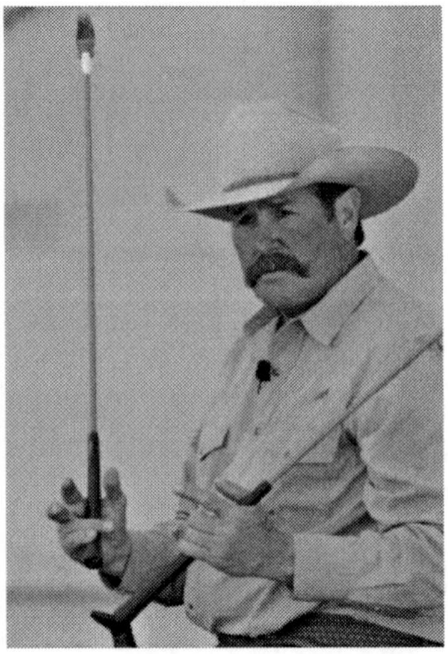

Figure 4.

Boredom

When we consider that horses only sleep 3 hours a day and play dominance games all day long, boredom becomes a huge issue that must be overcome during rehabilitation. The genetic makeup of horses has provided them with a huge play drive so that the smartest, strongest, and best puzzle solvers can establish themselves as leaders to ensure the survival of the species. When we take these games away from horses during their waking hours, boredom becomes exponential.

Boredom can lead to a variety of dysfunctional behavior patterns. Introverted horses will internalize and withdraw into themselves, while extroverted horses will externalize and attempt to interact with animals, people, or objects around it. Introverted horses are often misunderstood by handlers and thought to be "calm" because they are not always moving their feet or attempting to interact with the various animate and inanimate components of their environment. Introverted horses can become skeptical of handlers rapidly if they are bullied or treated roughly, this can lead to a horse that is likely to bolt or explode and is dangerous to interact with. Likewise extroverted horses are likely to try to dominate or disrespect caregivers and as a result are hard to deal with. Introverted horses require a lot of retreat from their handlers, i.e., they should wait until the horse relaxes and starts breathing regularly again before proceeding.

On a daily basis some mental stimulation in the form of a radio, a window, a companion, or a friendly groom is valuable. Extroverted horses require physical activity to overcome boredom – they have to be doing something at all times. Toys like large balls or frequent walks or other forms of physical activities like basic ground schooling are very important to an extroverted horse, and if they cannot move their feet, giving them something they can mouth and chew on or flip around will help. Displaced behaviors caused by the inability to move their feet can be alleviated in this way.

Isolation

Isolation is very stressful to horses and often results in many forms of dysfunctional behavior patterns. Pacing, weaving, popping lips, and fretting are secondary to anxiety caused by separation from other horses. To a horse isolation equals danger because the security of the herd is removed. If a horse cannot rejoin the herd anxiety levels can become so great that dysfunctional behavior patterns are established that are not easily overcome. Isolation is not an all or none condition. What may constitute isolation for one horse may not be for another. Some extremely dominant extroverted horses feel isolated if they cannot interact with all horses in their immediate surroundings. Other horses that are less dominant require less interaction. Also horses become accustomed to a certain amount of interaction. If this amount is either increased or decreased it represents an emotional stress for the individual. It is therefore important to consider the level of interaction that an individual has become accustomed to and try to mimic that in a rehabilitation situation. In all instances some form of companion must be provided for horses that are confined. This can be a mini, a donkey, a goat, or another horse.

Confinement

Confinement is another unnatural situation and can be very stressful. Indications that a horse is not coping with confinement are loss of appetite and depression. Different individuals seem to deal with confinement differently. Horses that are used to stall confinement deal with this better than individuals that have never been confined. Horses that have never been confined should be introduced to this situation prior to surgery if possible. It would be ideal to acclimate the horse to a stall and a new companion for a few hours/day for several days before surgery so that this situation will not constitute an unfamiliar environment post operatively. Horses that have been handled a lot as foals do much better in stall confinement situation because they do not perceive people and stall confinement as a threat. They can tolerate stressful situations without developing dysfunctional behavior patterns or becoming depressed. The most important time period is the first 168 hours (1 week) of life. The other very important time for socialization is the next 155 days (5 months). This concept has been clearly described by Dr. Miller in another segment of this chapter.

Environment and Experiences

Whenever possible the postoperative or post injury environment should mimic the conditions the horse has been accustomed to prior to surgery or injury. Some horses are much more relaxed and comfortable when turned out. Others seem to relax more in a confined area. These differences are in part due to different personality characteristics but also they are a function of previous learned adaptations and confidence levels. It might be difficult to predict which form of environment is best suited to an individual without previous knowledge obtained from the handler before surgery. Often it is mandatory that horses be confined to an unfamiliar environment for a certain time period after surgery or injury. This time should be kept to a minimum and the horse returned to its usual environment or a similar one as soon as possible.

Because horses are a precocial species that are full faculty learners from birth, they learn very quickly how to categorize things as safe or potentially harmful. What they have experienced in the past directly affects how they will potentially react in the future.

Pain

The level of pain that a horse can withstand is difficult to predict and not necessarily correlated with its innate horsenality. Usually, extroverted horses will react by constant motion or overt aggression while introverted horses will become withdrawn and freeze with fear… then explode violently. In all instances pain should be kept to a minimum because it is a huge stress riser and as such extremely detrimental to healing and the overall well being of the animal. Often times the best trained, most responsive, and highest level of performance horses are the least tolerant of pain. It is this personality characteristic that has allowed them to achieve the fine tuning necessary to succeed in competition.

Horses learn very quickly what happens before what happens actually happens. Essentially, this means we need to recognize what we do or don't do as a pattern prior to performing certain tasks. This is particularly true with tasks that are potentially painful or simply perceived by the horse as potentially painful. It takes approximately 7 times for a horse to start doing a positive behavior and only three times for a horse to perfect a flight reaction or negative behavior based on fear and adrenaline. Creating a truly positive reaction and partnership type behavior may take 30 times or more before it is truly a consistent pattern. That's 10 times longer than it takes to create a negative reaction. Our goal should be to prepare horses physically, mentally and emotionally prior to experiencing pain as well as preparing them to be better able to cope when actually experiencing pain.

Staff

When selecting the appropriate staff to be care givers to injured horses there are serious considerations that stem from fundamental horsemanship skills. Firstly, all care givers should be compassionate individuals. Beyond this, horsemen can be placed in one of three categories.

The first category is the naturally gifted horsemen also referred to as the "innate horseman". This individual somehow just knows what to do, when to do it, where to do it, and when to quit doing it. It is best to just stay out of their way and let them interact with the horse. These kinds of people will achieve the highest level of horsemanship skills and their potential is basically unlimited.

Next, there is the "learn it" kind of horseman. This individual is extremely motivated and will soak up everything that is thrown at him/her. This kind of person will achieve a high level of horsemanship skills but never as high as the "innate" horsemen. The third type of individual is not a horseman at all but the kind of individual that will bring out dysfunctional behavior in any horse, the "agitator". Many of these behaviors are hard to correct and they seem to get worse the longer this kind of person is around the horse. The major problem with this kind of individual is that he/she does not know their limitations. When they go beyond their limitations things usually go bad and the harder they try the worse things get. These people can only interact with a very few kinds of equine horsenality types or put in simpler terms - only a very few horses. The best horsemen can read a horse's horsenality and instinctively know what to do to form a partnership with that individual horse. Without the partnership the level of performance for both horse and human is very limited. The very best horsemen are the best puzzle solvers. They view their interactions with horses as games or puzzles to be solved. Therefore, the best puzzle solver is the best horsemen. In times of stress the partnership they have formed will allow the two (horse and man) to solve the puzzle together no matter how stressful the situation or how intense the competition becomes.

Equine veterinary care givers must be evaluated not only by their medical knowledge but also by their horsemanship abilities. They should constantly strive to form a partnership with each patient realizing full well that no two equine patients are alike and no two rehabilitation situations will be completely alike. Horses achieve much higher adrenalin levels than humans and are also much more sensitive, skeptical, claustrophobic, and panicky. It is the partnership that the care giver forms with the equine patient that will allow that individual to successfully care for an injured or rehabilitating horse. They need to learn how to read horse behavior at the most subtle levels, to know when to approach or when to retreat, have the patience to ask and wait for permission to approach, and to leave things on a good note – which may mean staying with the horse until it is relaxed after administering a treatment, or desensitizing the treated area. In setting things up for success, sometimes what you do after you did what you had to do is the key.

SPECIFIC CONSIDERATIONS OF BICEPS
CASSIE SMITH

Boredom

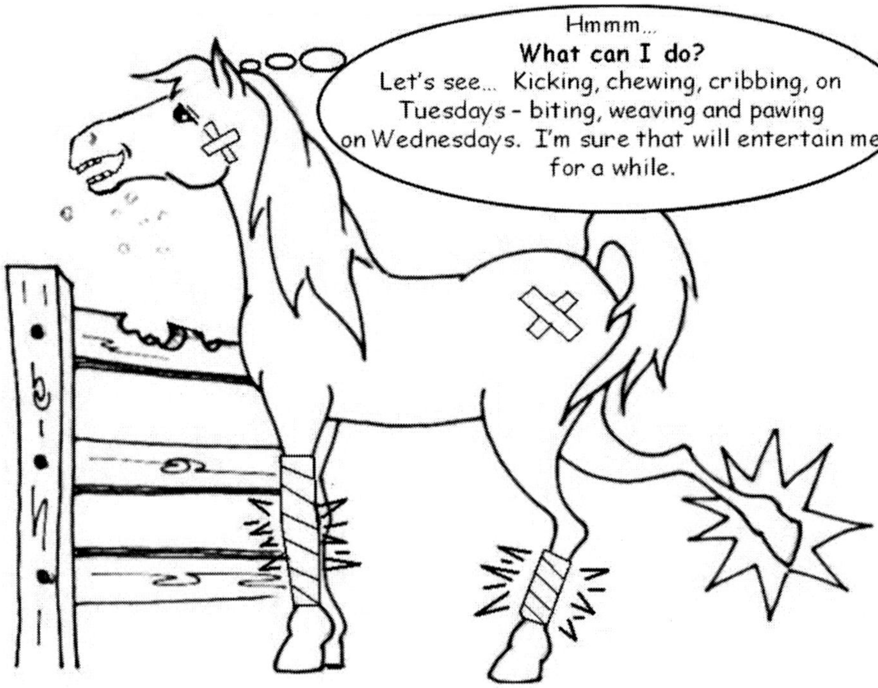

Figure 5.

Observe and gather information about this particular horse that will assist in preventing boredom for this particular horse (Figure 5).

Determine if horse is introvert or extrovert in order to determine if mental or physical stimulation will be primarily focused on.

Design stall, pen or turnout area in a manner that allows creative ways to safely approach, retreat and interact with patient.

Plan activities and environments for physical and/or mental stimulation as needed, utilizing toys, sounds, smells, interaction, etc.

Treat each horse as an individual and unique puzzle in order to think creatively and possibly differently on a daily basis.

Have compassionate, skilled and knowledgeable horseman on hand to advise and interact with the horse's physical, mental and emotional needs during rehabilitation.

BOREDOM.

Do		**Don't**
Utilize safe toys.	⟷	Don't leave toys so long that they are no longer interesting.
Allow horse to have play area large enough for safe movement.	⟷	Don't assume smaller areas prevent safe movement and exercise.
Provide multiple sensory stimulation, such as radio for sound, unique smells and tastes, such as apple cider vinegar, molasses, garlic, sage, mint, etc. strategically placed to create curiosity.	⟷	Don't use tastes or smells that can't be safely ingested if licked or swallowed.
Spend time with horse grooming, playing on line or at liberty, practicing simulated medical care to build confidence, curiosity and trust.	⟷	Don't make this time more about training and obedience – this time is for building a relationship and a partnership.

Isolation

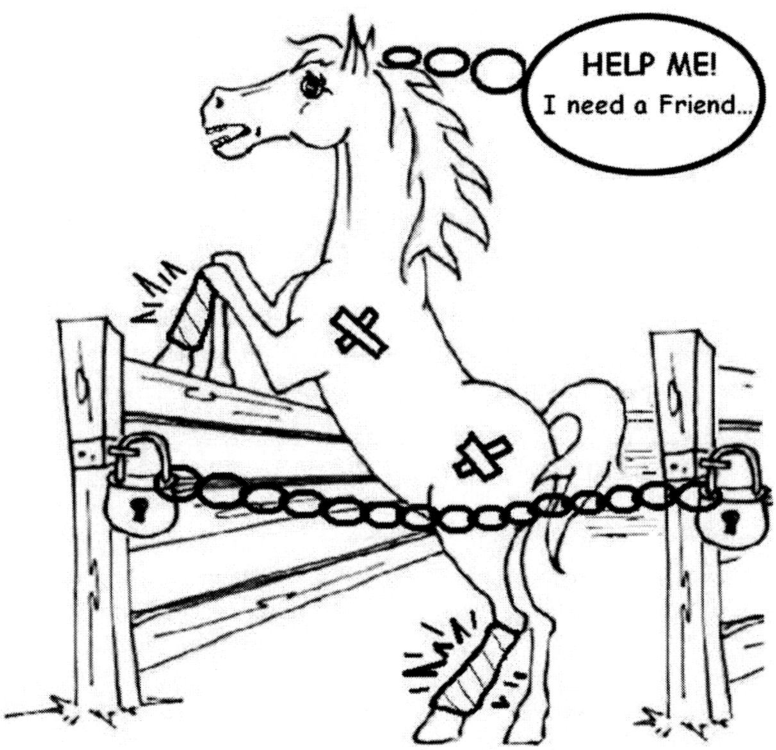

Figure 6.

Make prior and proper preparations for a companion (donkey, mini, horse or goat) to be introduced and at hand before and after medical procedures (Figure 6).

Observe patient and the degree of concern they express outwardly or inwardly to determine the stress level they are experiencing.

Experiment with types and quantity of companions necessary to eliminate isolation concerns.

ISOLATION.

Do		Don't
Have facility designed for safe interaction with a companion/companions.	↔	Don't put patient or companion in a position where they can be harmed.
Select companions that are easy to work with and get along well with others.	↔	Don't assume all smaller companions such as goats, minis or donkeys are always suitable companions.
Be prepared for patient to still express concerns regarding isolation even with a companion.	↔	Don't rule out turning the horse out with a herd in a large safe area if extreme isolation stress is obvious.

Confinement

Inquire about the past history of the patient and what has been normal for them.

Recognize that for some horses, small stall confinement will create more problems than it prevents. Various sizes of turnout areas may be necessary for optimal rest and relaxation of certain individuals (Figure 7).

Don't assume that small areas limit or prevent excessive physical and mental activity. Again, prior and proper preparation would be advised for horses that are not accustomed to stall confinement or even horses that are simply not comfortable in new surroundings.

Do		Don't
Observe patient's reaction to being confined daily.	↔	Don't assume patient's initial calm demeanor will remain as multiple medical procedures are performed.
Have flexibility in providing varying sizes of turnouts and stalls.	↔	Don't always assume larger areas will cause patient to be more prone to injury.

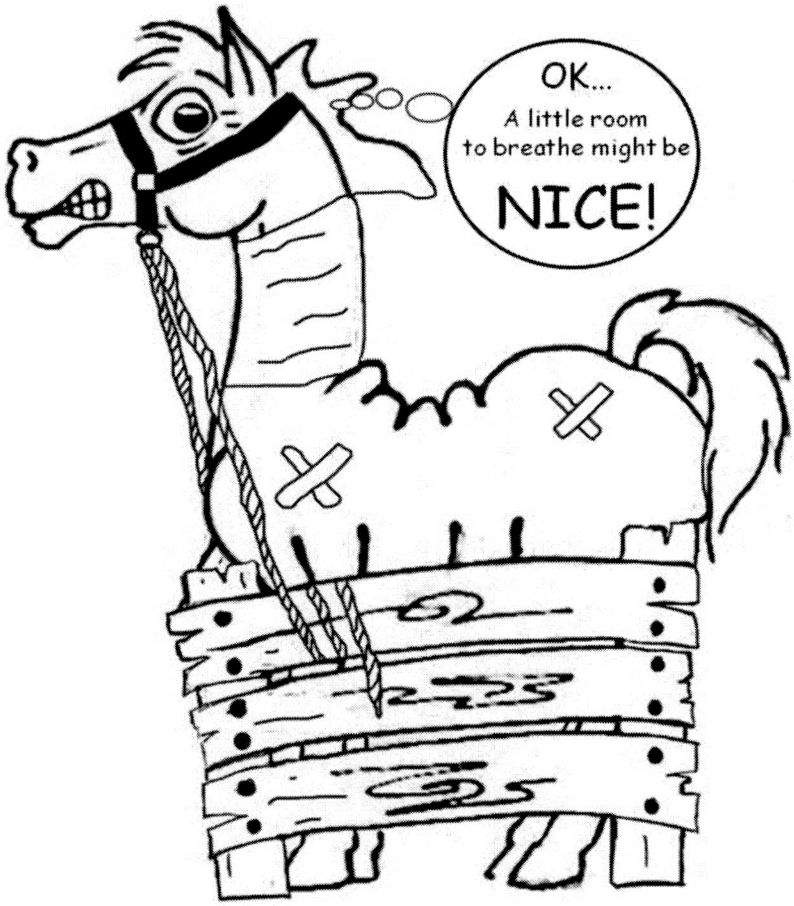

Figure 7.

CONFINEMENT

By preparing in advance to serious medical procedures you can greatly enhance the outcome both physically, mentally and emotionally.

Environment and Experiences

Once more, inquire about the past history of the patient and what has been normal for them.

Ultimately though, trust the horse and what he tells us. Observe reactions to determine how the horse perceives all situations. This will allow you to predict the likely outcomes during pre-op and post-op activities.

If rough handling or pain has been the pattern in the past they will come to expect all procedures to have the same outcome (Figure 8).

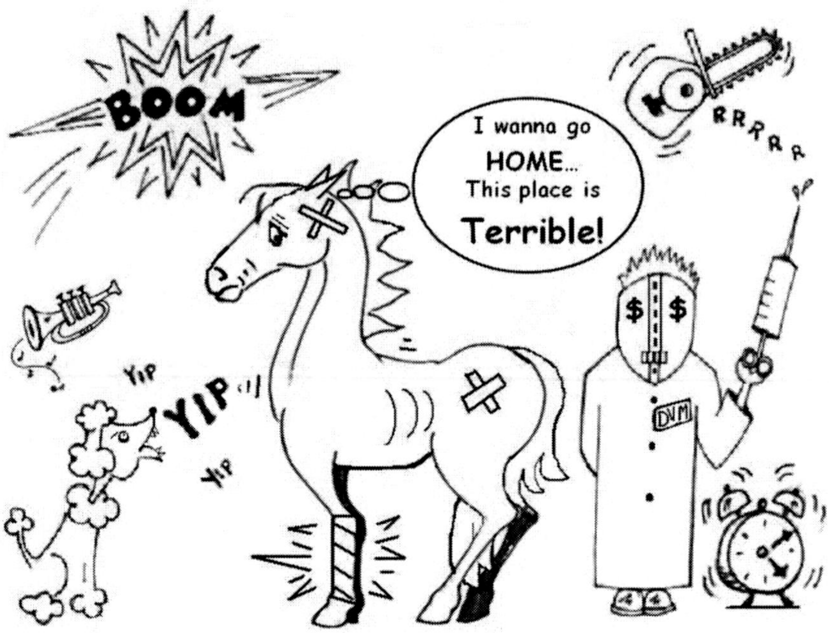
BOOM
I wanna go
HOME...
This place is
Terrible!
RRRRR
YIP
YIP
YIP
DVM

Figure 8.

Our goal should be to properly prepare the horse so that their expectations are changed.

If on the other hand they have experienced prior and proper preparation you can expect the rehabilitation process to be less stressful and certainly have more opportunity for success (Figure 9).

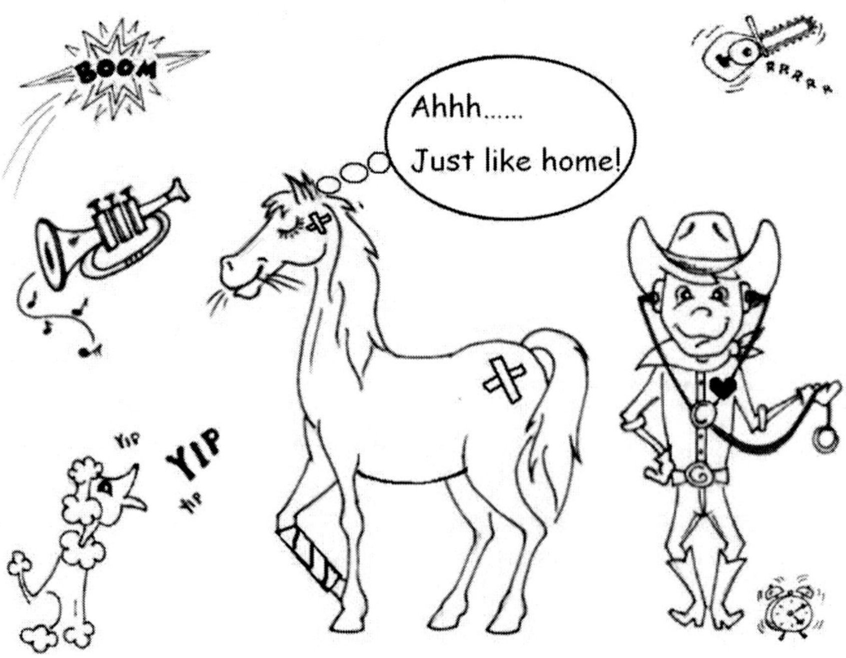
BOOM
Ahhh......
Just like home!
RRRRR
YIP
YIP
YIP

Figure 9.

ENVIROMENT and EXPERIENCES.

Do		Don't
Inquire about patient's history with regards to life experience with vets, new locations and new environments.	↔	Don't let patient's history be your primary source for determining the probable reactions to care and procedures.
Observe and compare patient's demeanor and degree of cooperation with what you have been told in order to develop strategies for overall care.	↔	Don't create more problems with difficult patients by allowing inexperienced or agitator type caregivers to interact with horses that are unconfident, stressed, inexperienced, extremely anxious or combative.
Create rehabilitation programs that promote confidence, curiosity, sensitivity and dignity for the horse.	↔	Don't do things to the horse without recognizing and understanding what their perspective on that task is. Remember - they don't think we are to going to hurt them– they think we are going to kill them.
Ask permission before barging in on horse's environment/stall. Extend hand – let them approach you instead of immediately trying to catch or halter the horse.	↔	Don't assume a quiet or inactive horse is not stressed or concerned by your approach or procedure.
Create expectations of something positive more often than something negative.	↔	Don't always enter environment/stall with the intention of doing something to the horse

Pain

Managing pain (Figure 10) will vary with each individual horse. By utilizing effective horsemanship techniques that minimize stress or anxiety we can be more confident that any medications used will have a better opportunity of being more effective or perhaps even unnecessary.

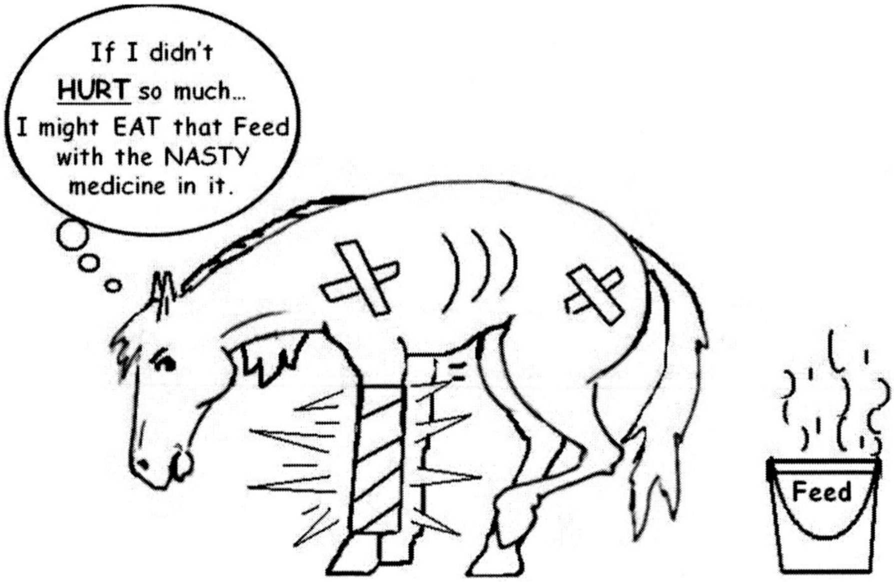
If I didn't
HURT so much...
I might EAT that Feed
with the NASTY
medicine in it.
Feed

Figure 10.

PAIN

Do		Don't
Take time to simulate procedures in a manner that prepares the patient to have confidence and trust even if something is painful. Reward positive behavior with treats, rubs, scratches, or simply retreat from the horse.	↔	Don't ignore mild reactions to routine procedures. If reaction is continually ignored it will likely escalate to extreme as time goes on.
Recognize that each painful procedure should be followed up with something that is clearly positive from the horse's perspective.	↔	Don't create patterns of negative expectations by performing unpleasant tasks routinely.
Change routine prior to and after routinely unpleasant tasks. Recognize that even cooperative patients <u>may</u> be experiencing extreme anxiety that is not outwardly expressed at the time of procedure.	↔	Don't forget to utilize <u>approach and retreat</u> techniques in all interactions with the patient. Taking a little more time initially will prevent escalated and dangerous situations in the future.

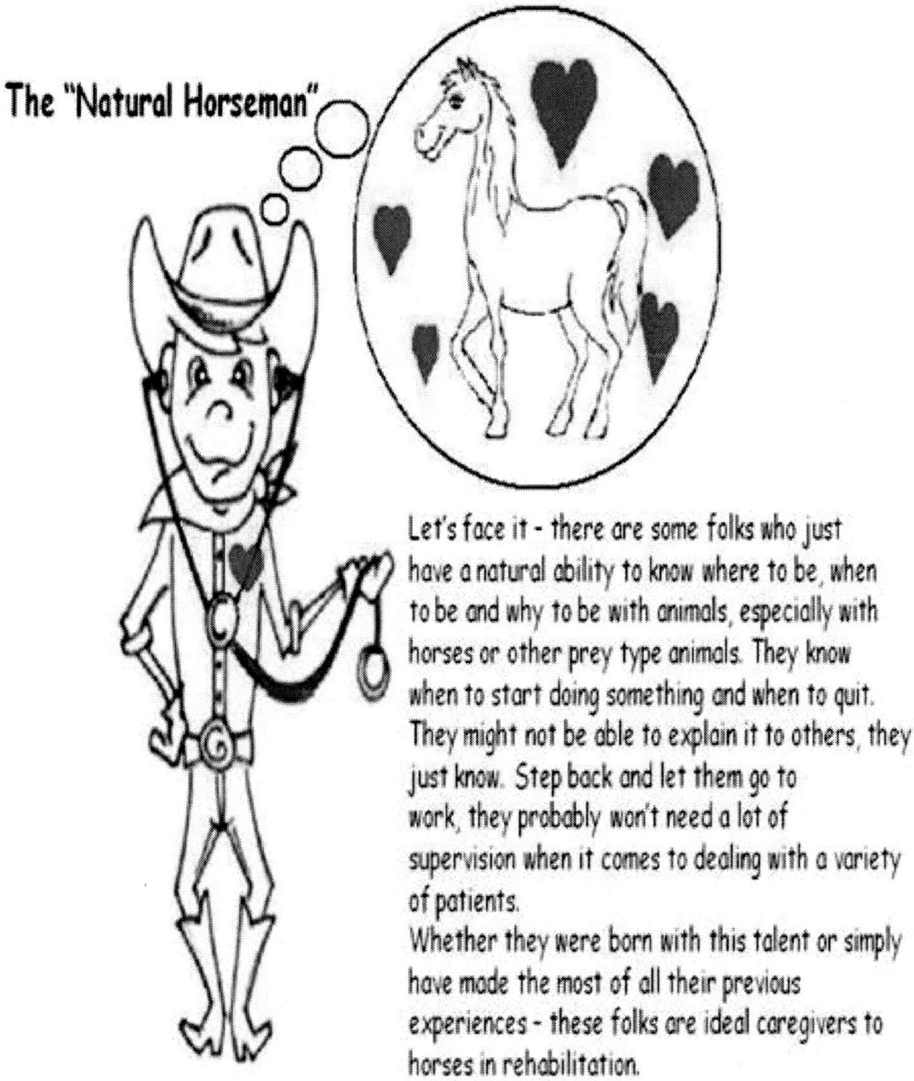
The "Natural Horseman"
Let's face it - there are some folks who just have a natural ability to know where to be, when to be and why to be with animals, especially with horses or other prey type animals. They know when to start doing something and when to quit. They might not be able to explain it to others, they just know. Step back and let them go to work, they probably won't need a lot of supervision when it comes to dealing with a variety of patients.
Whether they were born with this talent or simply have made the most of all their previous experiences - these folks are ideal caregivers to horses in rehabilitation.

Figure 11.

Staff

Because each horse has their own level of pain tolerance, degree of confidence, and experience, we should take the time to analyze each horse before assuming a fixed method for treating pain or assumed pain. Additionally, caregivers should be able to recognize when a horse has a fear of any procedure that he assumes will be painful. Routine simple tasks such as administering shots, monitoring temp and heart rate can bring on extreme reactions if performed in a manner that is considered by the horse as predatory. Slow down and take the time to ask permission before performing routine tasks. Horses are very quick to learn if we are a potential threat. This is influenced by our ability to appropriately use approach and retreat techniques. Predators do not retreat.

Clearly, this aspect of the BICEPS formula for success is the most critical of all. The individuals who will be responsible for the rehabilitation success or failure must be willing and able to learn how to treat more than the injury.

Some people have a natural talent and feel for what to do, when to do it, why to do it and when to quit (Figure 11).

For others they have to take the time that it takes to learn it so it will take them less time in the future to get it right (Figure 12).

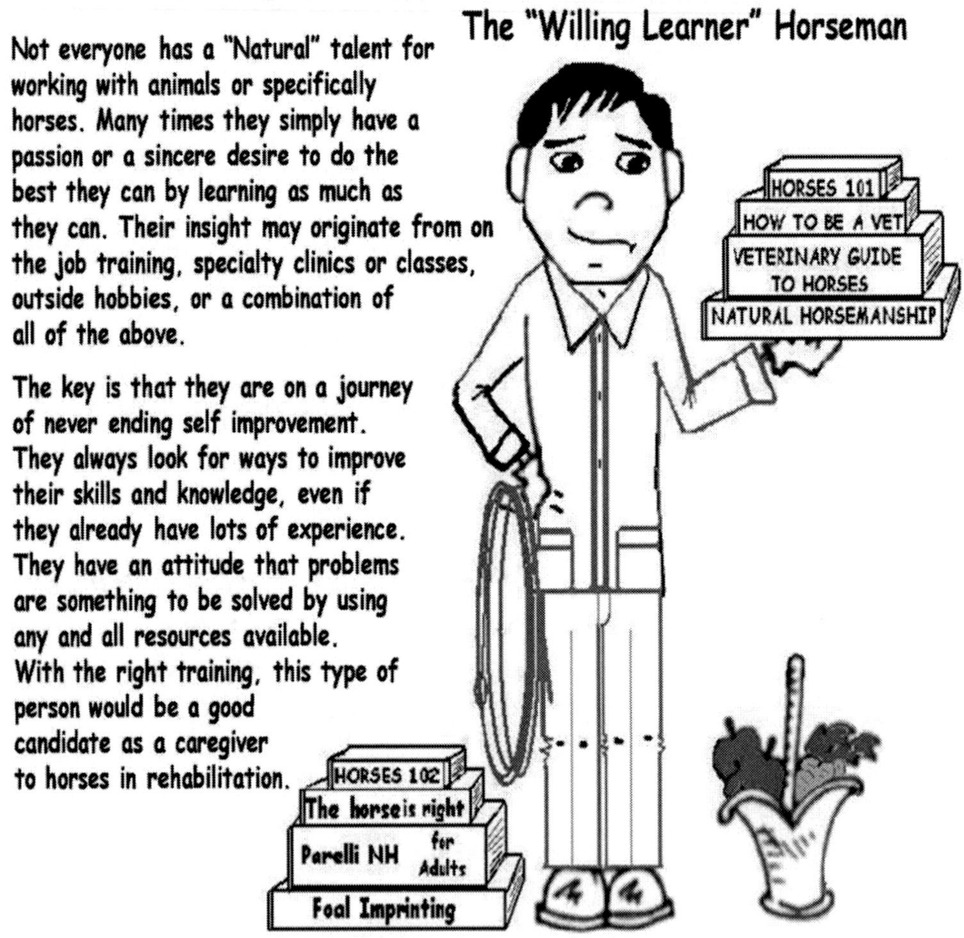

Figure 12.

Sadly the third category has very limited natural talent and the attitude of believing they are always right and the horse is always wrong. They have no idea of what they don't know and don't care to know. These individuals will probably demonstrate this aspect of their personality in areas beyond dealing with horses and should therefore be recognized as not suitable as a caregiver of a horse in rehabilitation (Figure 13).

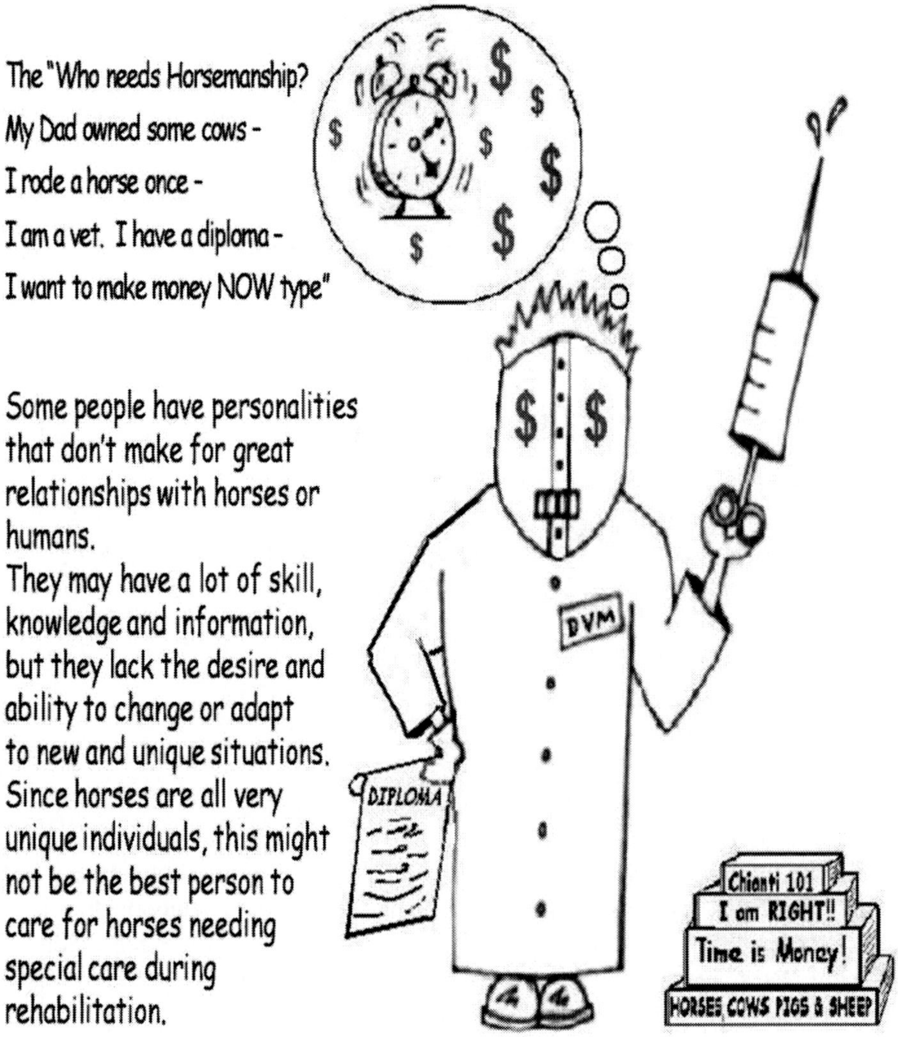

Figure 13.

One of the easiest ways to start the process of learning to be puzzle-solvers with horses is learning to think in terms of the opposite of normal. By simply recognizing what is normally thought of as always correct with horses and then considering what the opposite of that would be, we will likely find a more natural approach to our horsemanship skills. This can be proven time and time again when we consider how horses think, act and play. Many of the routine tasks we normally do to horses are extremely predatory. The same tasks can be accomplished by approaching them with and for the horse, utilizing skills that communicate our desires more naturally. In doing this, we can develop first a relationship and ultimately a partnership during the rehabilitation process. The most effective and consistent success of rehabilitation will require caregivers who are willing to learn how to treat more than the injury and physical needs of the equine patient.

Staff

Do		Don't
Make basic natural horsemanship training a part of the education process for all veterinarians, grooms, techs, and caregivers.	⟷	Don't assume all individuals with previous horse experience are ideal individuals as caregivers.
Recommend the study of natural horsemanship to the owners of horses in rehabilitation.	⟷	Don't expect everyone to want to learn anything different from what they already know.
Recommend foal imprinting for individuals involved with newborns that are expected to have any type of future interaction with humans.	⟷	Don't create problems by placing "agitator" type personalities in the position of caring for horses in rehabilitation.

Conclusion

In conclusion, the true success of long term rehabilitation of injured horses requires much more than the very best medical care available. The study of equine behavior, foal imprinting and natural horsemanship will dramatically improve the success of rehabilitating injured horses. In many cases, we can reduce or even eliminate post surgical trauma as well as prevent a variety of dysfunctional behavior patterns caused by long-term rehabilitation. The additional safety benefits to caregivers and patients only add to the sound reasoning for treating more than injuries.

The current revolution in horsemanship and dramatic success of natural horsemanship concepts, philosophies, principles and techniques gives us the opportunity for greatly improved care of horses worldwide. More and more owners of horses who are studying and implementing natural horsemanship will come to expect this skill and knowledge from their veterinarians, farriers and other individuals who provide care for their equine partners.

As professionals dedicated to caring for horses, our desire for successful rehabilitation should encompass more than successful surgeries and physically sound horses. Our goals should include learning how to recognize and treat the emotional and psychological needs of the horses we are caring for so that they return to fully functional lives free from anxiety, stress, or physical injury created by the rehabilitation process.

RECOMMENDED STUDY

Miller, R. M., & Close, P. (2003). *Imprint training of the newborn foal.* Colorado Springs, Colo.: Western Horseman Magazine.

Miller, R. M., & Lamb, R. A. (2005). *The revolution in horsemanship : and what it means to mankind.* Guilford, Conn.: Lyon's Press.

Miller, R. M. (2007). *Natural horsemanship explained: from heart to hands.* Guilford, CT: Lyons.

Miller, R. M. (1999). *Understanding the ancient secrets of the horse's mind.* Neenah, WI: Russell Meerdink Co.

Parelli, P., Kadash, K., & Parelli, K. (2003). *Natural horse-man-ship.* Colorado Springs, CO: Western Horseman Magazine.

Parelli Natural Horsemanship Program Linda and Pat Parelli www.parelli.com

Cartoons courtesy of Landon Pulley Laurel, MS and Cassie Smith OKC, OK

INDEX

A

B

C

D

G

H

I

J

K

L

M

P

Q

R

S

T

U

V

W

Y

Z